Clinical Observation
A Guide for Students in Speech, Language, and Hearing

Georgia Hambrecht, PhD, CCC-SLP
Professor
Department of Communication Sciences and Disorders
Western Carolina University
Cullowhee, North Carolina

Tracie Rice, AuD, CCC-A
Clinical Director
Department of Communication Sciences and Disorders
Western Carolina University
Cullowhee, North Carolina

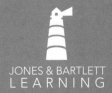

JONES & BARTLETT
LEARNING

World Headquarters

Jones & Bartlett Learning	Jones & Bartlett Learning	Jones & Bartlett Learning
40 Tall Pine Drive	Canada	International
Sudbury, MA 01776	6339 Ormindale Way	Barb House, Barb Mews
978-443-5000	Mississauga, Ontario L5V 1J2	London W6 7PA
info@jblearning.com	Canada	United Kingdom
www.jblearning.com		

Jones & Bartlett Learning books and products are available through most bookstores and online booksellers. To contact Jones & Bartlett Learning directly, call 800-832-0034, fax 978-443-8000, or visit our website, www.jblearning.com.

Substantial discounts on bulk quantities of Jones & Bartlett Learning publications are available to corporations, professional associations, and other qualified organizations. For details and specific discount information, contact the special sales department at Jones & Bartlett Learning via the above contact information or send an email to specialsales@jblearning.com.

The authors, editor, and publisher have made every effort to provide accurate information. However, they are not responsible for errors, omissions, or for any outcomes related to the use of the contents of this book and take no responsibility for the use of the products and procedures described. Treatments and side effects described in this book may not be applicable to all people; likewise, some people may require a dose or experience a side effect that is not described herein. Drugs and medical devices are discussed that may have limited availability controlled by the Food and Drug Administration (FDA) for use only in a research study or clinical trial. Research, clinical practice, and government regulations often change the accepted standard in this field. When consideration is being given to use of any drug in the clinical setting, the health care provider or reader is responsible for determining FDA status of the drug, reading the package insert, and reviewing prescribing information for the most up-to-date recommendations on dose, precautions, and contraindications, and determining the appropriate usage for the product. This is especially important in the case of drugs that are new or seldom used.

Production Credits

Publisher: David Cella
Associate Editor: Maro Gartside
Senior Production Editor: Renée Sekerak
Associate Production Editor: Jill Morton
Marketing Manager: Grace Richards
Manufacturing and Inventory Control
  Supervisor: Amy Bacus

Composition: Shawn Girsberger
Cover Design: Scott Moden
Cover Image: © Frank Anusewicz/ShutterStock, Inc.
Printing and Binding: Malloy Incorporated
Cover Printing: Malloy Incorporated

Library of Congress Cataloging-in-Publication Data
Hambrecht, Georgia.
  Clinical observation : a guide for students in speech, language, and hearing / by Georgia Hambrecht and Tracie Rice.
     p. cm.
  Includes bibliographical references and index.
  ISBN-13: 978-0-7637-7651-0
  ISBN-10: 0-7637-7651-3
  1. Speech disorders—Diagnosis. 2. Language disorders—Diagnosis. 3. Hearing disorders—Diagnosis. 4. Speech therapy. I. Rice, Tracie. II. Title.
  RC423.H3245 2011
  616.85'506—dc22
                    2010011838

6048
Printed in the United States of America
14 13 12 11 10   10 9 8 7 6 5 4 3 2 1

To our families

Contents

Acknowledgments

The Myron L. Coulter Faculty Center for Excellence in Teaching and Learning at Western Carolina University and the Center for Instruction, Research and Technology at Indiana State University have been instrumental in providing new ideas and encouragement for the continued development of our teaching philosophies and practices. We feel fortunate to have had training opportunities provided by these centers. We also wish to thank Sydney and Olivia for being a part of this endeavor.

Introduction

PURPOSE

This text is written for the pre-clinical or early clinical student in speech-language pathology to provide focus to the observation hours (a minimum of 25 hours) required by the American Speech-Language-Hearing Association for certification. It can be used as part of a class in observation/clinical processes or as a self-guide to the observation process. All those involved in the training, whether as teacher or learner, want relevant and meaningful experiences. This text will give a clear direction for guided observations so learners will have a better idea of what they may be observing, why it is relevant, and how observations serve as a building block to their future roles as clinicians.

INTRODUCTION

While observing holistically and discovering what catches your attention can be appropriate, 25 hours of unfocused observation may not be making the most of this valuable learning opportunity. This text presents worksheets to use as you carry out your hours of clinical observation. Each worksheet is organized under three headings. Heading 1, "The Focus," provides a brief knowledge snippet addressing one aspect of the clinical process. The focus is not meant to provide all the background available but rather to briefly highlight information you have learned in your prior courses. Heading 2, "The Activity," presents the assignments you as observer are to complete. This may be a series of questions to answer, checklists to complete, or charts to construct. Answers are provided for self-check where appropriate. Heading 3, "The Wrap-Up," encourages reflection and prediction based on your observation and activity completion. This section is a lot like journaling. You are asked to consider what you discovered during the observation and how you predict those discoveries will influence you in your quest to become a speech-language pathologist (SLP). It is also the place to connect what you are seeing with the knowledge you have gained from classes, textbooks, and journal articles.

Activities may be completed more than once, and more than one activity can be completed for an observation. A variety of observations are needed to complete all the activities across the big nine areas of practice. However, it is also good to view the same clinician-client(s) working together several times to get a better idea of routines, change over time, and building of relationships. An observation log sheet is provided at the end of the book (see Appendix A) for a convenient way to keep track of your observational hours and the chapters you have completed

POINT OF VIEW

There are several convictions that influenced the development of this book. First and foremost is our commitment to developing intentional learners. The National Panel report by the Association of American Colleges and Universities in *Great Expectations: A New Vision for Learning as a Nation Goes to College* (2002) emphasized the need to educate students in the twenty-first century to be intentional learners—empowered, informed, and responsible. Among the nine skills that the National Panel identified as areas in which the empowered learner excels is, "deriving meaning from experience, as well as gathering information from observation" (p. 22). It is this skill base that each chapter of this book aims to build and support. Culminating in the final chapter, "Your Turn," which directs each learner to take the chapter template and devise his or her own focus, activities, and reflection prompts and thus demonstrate his or her ability to be truly independent intentional observers, the completion of the book is not the finish but instead a start.

Second is our belief that the significant learning needed to prepare students *to do* speech, language, and hearing therapy must extend beyond content information. Clearly a knowledge base is vital but not sufficient in and of itself. L. Dee Fink (2003) identified his taxonomy for significant learning. Fink includes the dimensions of foundational knowledge, application, integration, human dimension, caring, and learning how to learn as the building blocks for teachers aiming to promote significant learning. Our chapters each begin with a reminder of knowledge-based material the learners have encountered in previous courses and then extends that knowledge to an application they complete during the observation. The reflection questions lead the learners to explore components of the remaining dimensions and to connect the observation to their individual past experiences and future desires.

Third is our certainty that what we as speech, language, and hearing professionals do and how we do it sets us apart as members of a distinct discipline. This discipline includes unique areas of practice reflected in "The Big Nine Areas" and "Supplemental Areas" sections and unique methods of practice reflected in "The Therapy Process" chapters. As Ehren (2000) noted in her article contrasting language classroom teaching with language classroom therapy, "therapy is a very specific, more intensive type of intervention, requiring focused expertise of the provider ..." (p. 221). The chapters introduce the learners to points of focus to center the development of their clinical expertise.

REFERENCES

The Association of American Colleges and Universities. (2002). *Great expectations: A new vision for learning as a nation goes to college.* Washington, DC: Association of Colleges and Universities.

Ehren, B. J. (2000). Maintaining a therapeutic focus and sharing responsibility for student success: Key to in-classroom speech-language pathologist in inclusive classrooms. *Language, Speech, and Hearing Services in Schools, 31,* 219–229.

Fink, L. D. (2003). *Creating significant learning experiences.* San Francisco, CA: Jossey-Bass.

Reviewers

Nancy D. Allen, MA, CCC-SLP
Clinical Director
Speech and Hearing Center
State University of New York at Plattsburgh

Catherine K. Bacon
Clinical Associate Professor
Department of Speech and Hearing Science
Arizona State University

Jill L. Brady, PhD, CCC-SLP
Assistant Professor
Department of Special Education and Clinical Services
Indiana University of Pennsylvania

Christine M. P. Cecconi, MA, CCC-SLP
Clinical Associate Professor and SLP Clinic Director
Department of Speech-Language Pathology and Audiology
Ithaca College

Rebekah F. Cunningham, PhD
Assistant Professor
Department of Audiology
Arizona School of Health Sciences
A.T. Still University

Claire M. Edwards, PhD, CCC-SLP
Assistant Professor
Department of Communication Science and Disorders
University of Montevallo

The Big Nine Areas

CHAPTER 1

Articulation

THE FOCUS

When dealing with articulation, it is important to note that there is a natural progression of sounds, meaning that certain sounds come easier when they are in a particular placement. It is easiest to obtain sounds in isolation, move to the syllable level (consonant plus vowel), then to words, phrases, sentences, and finally, conversation. A client would not be expected to move to the next level until mastery at the current level is obtained (typically 80 percent or greater). There are several methods of reaching articulation goals. The two methods that will be discussed in this chapter are moving in a systematic order, working on one sound at a time, and working on various sounds at the same time.

Within the word level, it is important to keep in mind the vocabulary initial, medial, and final. These placements are exactly what one would assume—initial at the beginning, medial in the middle, and final at the end of the word. Typically, when a client is ready to work on sounds at the word level, the initial placement is the easiest. The client can get the articulators in place in order to produce the sound. The clinician could come up with scenarios or other treatment activities to target the sound at the initial word placement with various vowel sounds following the target. The next step in the progression would be the final placement, and once that level is obtained, the medial position could be attempted.

The next method is working on various sounds at the same time. Rather than waiting until a client has obtained 80 percent accuracy at a certain position and then moving on to the next position, in this method, sounds in several positions or multiple sounds may be targeted at the same time. Using this method allows for more variation in activities and in some cases may allow the client to have mastery of more sounds faster than if he or she were to use the one-sound-at-a-time method.

It is important to keep in mind that articulation therapy is not always easy therapy. Many times the client gets bored or frustrated with trying to make the same sound over and over. The more opportunities for making the target sound correctly, the better, so be creative and come up with ways to incorporate the target sound into the entire session! One fabulous way of incorporating various activities is to use books in therapy. For instance, if a child is working on the /m/ sound, you could use the book, *If You Give a Moose a Muffin*. Do not stop with the book; make muffins with the child and take it another step by incorporating following directions and make use of the /m/ cooking words such as *mix* and *measure*. Make sure that your expectations for the client are realistic and that you are not concerned about sound corrections to errors that are not developmentally appropriate.

THE ACTIVITY

A. Crossword puzzle

Complete the crossword puzzle (**Figure 1–1**) using vocabulary learned in this chapter.

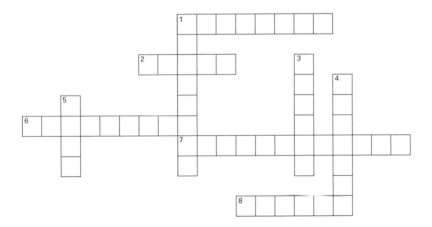

Figure 1–1 **Articulation Crossword Puzzle**

ACROSS
1. occurring as a CV (consonant plus vowel)
2. the end position in a word
6. the starting point for this type of articulation therapy
7. the final level for this type of articulation therapy
8. the last position to work on at the word level

DOWN
1. a complete thought (containing a subject and verb)
3. several 5 downs put together
4. the beginning part of a word
5. the step following 1 across

B. Important vocabulary

Define the vocabulary words provided and describe their relevance to the session you observed.

1. Initial:

_____

_____

_____

_____

2. Medial:

_____

_____

_____

_____

3. Final:

_____

_____

_____

_____

4. Isolation (with regard to sound):

_____

_____

_____

_____

AS YOU
OBSERVE...

C. Think about the client you just observed. Was one of the two methods described in this chapter used? If so, what method was used and what sounds were targeted? Develop an activity for the client you just observed that could be used with either method.

_____

_____

_____

_____

THE WRAP-UP

◻ Suggestions for Reflection

When working with sounds in isolation, clinicians use mirrors to view those sounds that are visible when being produced, tongue depressors to pinpoint location of tongue placement in the mouth, and verbal description of what the articulators are doing while the sound is being made. Complete **Table 1–1** on the sounds /s, f, p, and r/.

Table 1–1 Sound Teaching Technique Worksheet

Sound	Should a Mirror Be Used? If Yes, Specify What Would Be Viewed.	Should a Tongue Depressor Be Used? If Yes, Where Would It Touch?	Should Verbal Description Be Used? If Yes, Specify the Place of Production of the Sound.
/s/			
/f/			
/p/			
/r/			

Speculate on why the medial position is the final part to work on at the word level.

_____

_____

_____

_____

□ *Suggestions for Predictions*

How might therapy look different for a child versus an adult who may be working on the same sound?

_____

_____

_____

_____

Come up with an activity that could be used for a child (7 years old) working on the /l/ sound.

_____

_____

_____

_____

THE ANSWERS

A. Crossword puzzle

ACROSS
1. syllable
2. final
6. isolation
7. conversation
8. medial

DOWN
1. sentence
3. phrase
4. initial
5. word

B. Important vocabulary

1. Initial: Beginning
2. Medial: Middle
3. Final: Last
4. Isolation: The target sound produced alone or with no other sounds before or after the target sound.

CHAPTER 2

Fluency

THE FOCUS

Everyone experiences problems with fluency at some point in time. We may occasionally have trouble getting a word out (block), have long pauses either before or during a word (prolongation), repeat a sound or word several times (repetition), or even talk so fast that our words become jumbled. Each of these examples represents a type of dysfluency. When these types of problems occur often or in conjunction with facial grimaces or other instances of body tension, people may seek assistance with their fluency. There are many different treatment options when working with clients who are experiencing issues with fluency.

One overarching theme is to make sure that as a clinician you are giving the client time to complete his or her thoughts. It is often very difficult to do this because as communication partners, we become uncomfortable when someone is struggling to be fluent. We sometimes attempt to finish the sentence or thought for the person who is struggling so he does not have to work so hard to say what we assume he is trying to say. While this is often a natural inclination for most people, it is very important to remember not to do this. The client must learn techniques to use when she is experiencing problems with fluency, and if you are finishing thoughts for her, not only do you run the risk of her becoming frustrated, you are not allowing her to implement controls that have been learned.

In treatment, you may see the clinician and client talking about recent events or instances during which the person remembers struggling with fluency. Although the clinician may be engaging in conversation, he or she should be keeping data or recording the session for review. The number of dysfluencies and the controls used are examples of data points that are traditionally noted. The clinical supervisor may ask the clinician to keep other kinds of data as well.

As stated previously, there are many treatment methods to use with fluency. One method may be to teach the person how to use controls to move through a situation when he is not able to be fluent. Examples of controls include using easy onset speech—when you make sure you are relaxed (tongue, jaw, body) before beginning to speak, visualizing the word, and altering the rate or intensity of speech so the client learns control over his speech.

Another treatment option is to use delayed auditory feedback (DAF). Using this type of treatment, the client uses a device, which can be low-tech or high-tech, that allows her to hear her speech naturally as well as with a slight delay in what she said. Imagine hearing an echo but much faster than how you would normally hear that echo. This method gives the client additional auditory information that can sometimes aid in reducing the number of dysfluencies in a conversation. You may also see this in shared reading, where the client and the clinician are reading the same piece of information but the clinician is reading slightly slower than the client.

In fluency remediation, you want the client to experience the flow and feeling of fluent speech and DAF or choral reading can help provide this fluent experience. Fluency disorders may occur in children or adults. Generally, you will not observe a child earlier than age four or five. There are times in a preschooler's life when he goes through stages of normal dysfluency. These stages just mean that it is not out of the ordinary for a child around age 3 or 4 years old to have times when he repeats sounds or words. It may seem that the child is having fluency problems often, and many times this concerns parents or other adults in the child's life. Because these are normal stages, these children are typically not placed in therapy unless there are additional issues such as a high level of stress on the child's part about the fluency problem or the fluency problem being accompanied by facial grimaces or eye blinks. For the most part this stage passes by about age 5 or 6. When observing clients working on fluency, you will likely be seeing older children or adults.

Fluency treatment typically lasts for several years. The client may come in frequently to start and then change to only coming in once a week or even once a month for consultation. Sometimes these clients experience times when they seem to have more difficulty with fluency and may come in more often for assistance. There are many variables that can alter a person's fluency such as high stress, lack of sleep, and being in more demanding conversational situations. Fluency treatment does not follow the same course as other speech or language treatments that are discontinued once goals have been met. With speech problems such as articulation, when the client has mastered the skill, more often than not she does not need to continue therapy because she will not typically revert back to mispronouncing a sound she has learned to pronounce correctly. However, fluency is not something a person never has to deal with once he has reached his goals. As circumstances change, the rate of fluency may also change, thus requiring him to enroll in therapy again.

THE ACTIVITY

A. Rate the following scenarios using a 1 if the clinician is not assisting the client to learn techniques and a 2 if the clinician is assisting the client in learning techniques. Give your reasoning behind your rating.

Scenario 1. The client is talking about a class he is in and is being very fluent. He begins describing a situation that occurred yesterday and repeats the beginning sound in a word several times. The clinician sees the client is getting frustrated, and there is suddenly silence in the room. The clinician does not speak for about 45 seconds and then the client starts talking again about the situation that occurred in class.

Rating: ___

Reasoning: _____

_____

_____

_____

Scenario 2. The client and clinician are talking about their favorite restaurants. The clinician begins telling a story about something that happened the last time she went to her favorite restaurant. The client seems very interested and the clinician talks nonstop for over five minutes.

Rating: ___

Reasoning: _____

_____

_____

_____

Scenario 3. The clinician is reading with a client but seems to be a bit distracted today. During the shared reading, the clinician is reading at a pace much slower than the client. The client has finished the sentence before the clinician gets halfway through.

Rating: ____

Reasoning: _____

_____

_____

_____

Scenario 4. The clinician asks the client to describe a situation when the client has recently experienced several blocks in a conversation. The clinician can sense the tension in the client's voice and body language as the client begins to describe the situation. The clinician reminds the client about the controls that have been working for the client and then asks the client to finish her story.

Rating: ____

Reasoning: _____

_____

_____

_____

B. What are controls, and what controls have been discussed in this chapter?

_____

_____

_____

_____

C. What is blocking?

_____

_____

_____

_____

AS YOU
OBSERVE...

D. The typical client or common occurrences were described in the focus section but the client you are observing may or may not fit this typical pattern. Answer the following questions about the client with fluency issues and the therapy that you observed.

   1. Fluency type(s) observed:

Repetitions_____

_____

_____

_____

Prolongations_____

_____

_____

_____

Blocks_____

_____

_____

_____

   2. Grimaces or unusual body movements observed (please describe):

_____

_____

_____

_____

   3. Did the client's communication partner give the client time to complete his/her thoughts?

_____

_____

_____

_____

4. Controls taught or practiced:

_____

_____

_____

_____

5. Description of data taken:

_____

_____

_____

_____

6. Methods used to promote the experiencing of fluent speech:

_____

_____

_____

_____

7. Approximate age of client: _____

8. Age when this client was first seen in therapy: _____

THE WRAP-UP

◻ _Suggestions for Reflection_

In what ways was the client you observed unique? Is there a value in describing when each client will vary from that typical description in one or more ways?

_____

_____

_____

_____

While observing a fluency client, what types of dysfluency did you observe? Was this client successful in using controls? What controls did the client use?

_____

_____

_____

_____

Think back to a time when you have experienced problems with fluency. What were the conditions surrounding that particular conversation? Can you find a reason that you may have been dysfluent?

_____

_____

_____

_____

◻ *Suggestions for Prediction*

List ways in which you can communicate more effectively with someone who has problems with fluency.

_____

_____

_____

_____

As a clinician, how will you keep accurate data during a fluency session (review the data chapter)? What do you think will be the most difficult aspects of keeping data? What will be the most difficult aspects of working with a client with fluency problems? How might you encourage a client without talking for him?

_____

_____

_____

_____

ANSWERS

A.

Scenario 1. Rating 2: The clinician should give the client time to finish. In some instances, it will seem that a long time has passed before the client continues but the clinician does not want to finish the client's thoughts just to make it more comfortable for herself.

Scenario 2. Rating 1: The clinician should never be talking more than the client. Although the clinician must engage in the conversation, it is important to be more client focused.

Scenario 3. Rating 1: The clinician must remain focused during a session. With shared reading and delay auditory feedback, there is only a slight delay between what the client has read and what the clinician is reading.

Scenario 4. Rating 2: The clinician sensed the anxiety of the client. It is important to remind clients about the controls that have been working and encourage them to begin in a relaxed state.

B. Controls are techniques that a client uses to increase his or her fluency rate. Examples of controls discussed in this chapter include using easy onset speech, visualizing the word, and varying the rate or intensity of speech.

C. Blocking is when a person is trying to articulate a word but no sound is emitted.

CHAPTER 3

Voice

Your voice characteristics are so much a part of defining you as a unique individual. Friends identify you after hearing only a few words even over the phone. When voice disorders occur, remediation is essential. Voice disorders are often classified into the areas of loudness, quality, or pitch. The causes of all three categories of voice problems can be due to inappropriate use (functional causes) or structural damage or irregularities (organic causes). Most of us have experienced temporary voice problems in all three areas. Have you ever experienced loudness problems when you had laryngitis or a time that your voice was not as strong as it typically is and you felt as if you were straining just to be loud enough to be heard? Have you ever experienced quality problems when you had a bad cold with a blocked nasal cavity and had a denasal vocal quality (all your /m/s came out as /b/s)? Have you ever experienced pitch problems when your voice had pitch breaks or you spoke in a falsetto or unnaturally low voice?

When voice problems persist or result in pain or excessive throat clearing, the individual will seek professional help to return to normal or near normal vocal health. Before an SLP will begin treatment for a client with voice problems, the client will require medical clearance from a physician, most likely an ear, nose, and throat physician (otolaryngologist). This is done in order to make sure that there is no structural damage that should be taken care of before treatment begins or that certain therapies are not contraindicated. Some medical issues that may require further investigation and treatment by a doctor are vocal nodules, vocal polyps, paralyzed vocal fold(s), cancer of the larynx, reflux, or consistent drainage due to allergies. After medical clearance, the therapy may begin.

Voice therapy may consist of a variety of treatment options. Teaching the client to manage his voice by establishing healthy vocal habits is one component of voice therapy. If a client has the habit of talking too loudly or softly or talking in an inappropriate pitch or with insufficient breath support, the speech-language pathologist may help the client to identify times when he is using harmful vocal habits and substitute better ways of using his voice. It sometimes takes many reminders before the client can self-monitor. In these situations, it is important for the clinician to interject and give the client helpful hints on using better vocal habits. If a client does not stay hydrated and is in a position when she must talk a lot or use a louder voice (such as a teacher), the speech-language pathologist may help her come up with a plan to drink more water during the day to keep her throat moist or to employ a microphone to avoid straining her voice to be heard. Smoking, consumption of alcohol or caffeinated drinks, and straining the voice should be avoided and the client should be encouraged to practice good vocal hygiene.

Another common therapy technique is using computerized software such as the Computerized Speech Lab (CSL, KayPENTAX), which allows the client's voice to be recorded and the client to have a visual representation of his voice. The CSL has features that allow the client to see what pitch he typically uses, which can be compared to norms to see if he is speaking at a pitch that is too high or too low—either of those can cause vocal strain. The CSL also provides the option of seeing how long a client can sustain a certain sound (such as /a/) before his voice gives out. The CSL is a great tool that can be used so the client can not only hear his own progress but see the progress as well. Many of the software companies have games that are included in the software so the client is not just performing tasks and getting a visual picture of her voice, but she is able to participate in games that reinforce appropriate use of the voice. An example of a game that a 15-year-old client focusing on pitch modification enjoyed was the cat and mouse game on the CSL. In this game, the client must raise or lower her pitch in order to move the mouse across the screen to various pieces of cheese. A cat comes out to chase the mouse and the client has to raise or lower her voice faster and for longer periods of time to avoid the cat. While these games are great for kids, they are also enjoyable for many adults and provide them with a way to monitor their voice in a visual format. If the treatment facility does not have these types of computerized programs available, treatment can be done by tape recording the client in various situations and playing it back. Often times, the client cannot detect changes in his voice when it is happening, but if he hears himself in a recorded format, he can indicate when changes occurred and what may have been the cause of that change.

Some breathing techniques may be taught to clients with vocal problems as vocal support is a necessary component of voice production. Clients with Parkinson's disease often have a very breathy quality voice and speak very softly. These clients lose muscle tone and may have to learn to retrain their brain and body when speaking. Many times, these clients need to be taught how to take deep breaths and speak on the exhalation. The deeper breath they take, the more force they can use when speaking. Clients may have to take more breaths than they once did when speaking in order to help provide power to their voice.

Regardless, the type or cause of the voice problem, counseling will likely be a part of therapy to help the client embrace a modified vocal characteristic. Clinicians need to be sensitive to the personal identity aspect of this treatment and the difficulties involved in generalizing the gains made in therapy to all aspects of an individual's life.

THE ACTIVITY

A. Determine what the client is doing incorrectly and give recommendations to the client.

1. A client with a strained voice is in the waiting room talking to a family member. You want to see what progress the client is making with self-monitoring so you stand out of sight and listen to the conversation. You hear the family member ask the client a question and the client responds with a two-minute answer that starts out strong but quickly changes to a whispered voice.

_____

_____

_____

_____

2. It is 4:00 p.m., and you are asking the client what she has had to drink today. The client reports that she has had one cup of coffee and one 8-ounce can of soda.

_____

_____

_____

_____

3. You are getting ready to see a client who has been making progress and has been talking in his normal frequency (this particular client did not like the sound of his voice and he always tried

to use a lower frequency voice than was appropriate for him). The client called to say he was running late and you thought it was his dad calling.

_____

_____

_____

_____

B. Develop an activity to help an adult client who talks using a very high pitch. Explain the rationale for the activity to the client in sufficient detail. This client has been diagnosed with vocal nodules and the goal is to have the client be able to independently monitor her pitch and loudness level use in a typical conversation.

_____

_____

_____

_____

AS YOU
OBSERVE...
C. Answer the series of yes/no questions provided in **Table 3–1** concerning the voice session you are observing by putting a check in either the Yes or No column. For every Yes answer complete the last column by providing a detailed description with at least one specific example to support your Yes answer.

THE WRAP-UP

◻ *Suggestions for Reflection*

What factors make it so difficult for clients to get to a point where they can appropriately self-monitor and change their voice when needed?

_____

_____

_____

_____

Table 3–1 Voice Observation Checklist

Question	Answer Yes	Answer No	Description/Example if Answer Is Yes
1. Is the focus of remediation loudness?			
2. Is the focus of remediation pitch?			
3. Is the focus of remediation quality?			
4. Is the cause of the voice disorder functional?			
5. Is the cause of the voice disorder organic?			
6. Were healthy/ unhealthy vocal habits discussed?			
7. Was a visual display of the vocal output examined?			
8. Was an audio recording made and evaluated?			
9. Was a motivator/ reinforcer used?			
10. Was breath support monitored?			
11. Was a counseling focus evident?			
12. Was generalization of gains beyond the therapy room included?			

Identify a situation you have been in when you strained your voice. What were you doing? Did the vocal strain last or did it go away quickly? Did you do anything that helped your voice? If so what did you do? List some recommendations you could give a client with a hoarse voice.

_____

_____

_____

_____

◻ *Suggestions for Prediction*

Explain why it is important to get medical clearance before beginning treatment with voice clients. What do you do if a client refuses to see a doctor? Can you have him sign a waiver or would you refuse services? Why or why not?

_____

_____

_____

_____

List some reasons a child or teenager may have voice problems. Would your therapy differ from that for an adult? How would the therapy be different and why?

_____

_____

_____

_____

ANSWERS

A.

1. The client is not self-monitoring; you could record a conversation with the client and have him listen to it and critique himself. Note that using a whispered voice is not a good solution. Whispering does not decrease the strain put on the vocal folds.

2. The client is not staying hydrated. Help the client develop a log she will use to write down how much fluid she drinks every day for a week.

3. The client is not talking in his fundamental frequency outside therapy. Use the CSL or record the client using various pitches to see which one the client thinks is most appropriate. Help him to identify the frequency that is the best for him.

B. You and the client could read a magazine article and discuss it. Record the conversation and rate the conversation independently, then compare notes to see if the client is able to compare her voice to yours and identify times when she could have altered her voice or the conversation to accomplish her goal.

CHAPTER 4

Swallowing

THE FOCUS

Speech-language pathologists have not always worked with patients with swallowing disorders. Within the last 15 years, the American Speech-Language-Hearing Association recognized dysphagia (swallowing problems) as being a part of the scope of practice of a speech-language pathologist. SLPs not only deal with swallowing treatment but also diagnosing dysphagia. Primarily the diagnosis will be made in a hospital setting; however, in the past 5–10 years, SLPs have begun obtaining equipment and training in diagnosing patients. This has led to SLPs having portable equipment that allows them to view a person's throat while swallowing. This type of evaluation is known as FEES (flexible endoscopic evaluation of swallowing). Typically, this type of equipment does not show the full swallow (such as what may be seen when a person goes to a hospital setting for a barium swallow study); however, it does allow the SLP to view the throat in several different stages of the swallow.

There are many treatment options for persons with swallowing difficulty. Suggestions vary depending on the specific area of swallowing disorder and may include chewing food multiple times before swallowing, using a chin tuck when swallowing, using thickening agents in liquids, and doing strengthening exercises for swallow. Other methods may also be recommended as treatment methods, but those listed are some typical ones you see in a clinic setting. When asking a client to use a chin tuck, you are simply having the client tuck his chin to his chest before he swallows the bolus of food. This method sets the pharyngeal cavity up so the epiglottis covers the trachea and food does not escape into the lungs (or as an SLP would say, the patient does not experience aspiration). The clinician typically just reminds the client to tuck his chin before each swallow. This may take many reminders to begin with in hopes of the client remembering to do this on his own, thus keeping him safe during eating and being able to eat foods he enjoys. This method would not be recommended for clients who have significant swallow problems or have very weak muscles, such as patients with Parkinson's, as the chin tuck method may not provide enough protection.

There are various thickening agents that may be used. Some terms you may hear are *nectar thick*, *honey thick*, and *pudding thick*. Nectar thick is approximately the same consistency of apricot juice. Honey thick and pudding thick are what one would think, honey and pudding consistency. These thickening agents are used when a person has difficulty with swallowing liquids without aspirating. In order to keep clients hydrated, yet safe, these thickening agents may be added to liquid. These agents can be ordered by a client or her family members or in the case of a client in a long-term care facility, the facility staff would make sure the client had the proper consistency. The clinician may still work with the client on strengthening exercises, and in some cases a client may be able to safely stop using the thickening agents.

Some strengthening exercises may include strengthening the lips, tongue, and jaw by holding items such as a straw or piece of licorice in the mouth at the midline of the tongue and moving it to one side of the mouth and then the other. Another exercise includes having clients hold those same items or a tongue depressor in their mouth using the lips to hold tight to the object while the clinician tries to remove the object. Strengthening the lips, tongue, and jaw help a client to have better control over the bolus of food when moving the food through the oral stage (while it is in the mouth) to the pharyngeal stage (when it is going down the throat).

When you are the clinician working with clients who have dysphagia, it is important to remember that you may be responsible for educating the client and his family members on the disorders and the importance of following the recommendations. For most people, eating is an enjoyable part of life. When there is a disorder that causes a person to not be able to swallow normally or not be able to eat the foods she enjoys, she may experience depression and withdrawal. As a clinician you will need to be aware of these issues and work with the client and her family members to keep daily living as normal as possible while keeping eating safe.

THE ACTIVITY

A. Complete the data sheet in **Table 4–1** using this information: Chin tuck exercises—goal is client will independently use chin tuck before each swallow. Data—client used chin tuck five times when reminded verbally, three times when reminded by pointing to throat, and one time independently.

Table 4–1 Swallowing Activity Recording Form

Goal:

Verbal reminder:

Visual reminder:

Independent:

B. Think about the client you just observed. Develop a data sheet using the information you remember from one or two of the activities completed in the session.

C. Determine which treatment method discussed in this chapter is being used.

   1. The clinician is mixing a substance into the client's liquids.

   2. The client is putting her chin to her chest before swallowing.

   3. The clinician is pulling a tongue depressor out of the client's mouth.

4. The clinician is counting the number of times the client is chewing before the client is swallowing.

_____

_____

_____

_____

THE WRAP-UP

◻ *Suggestions for Reflection*

Think about the client you just observed. What were the client's greatest concerns about his difficulty swallowing? Was there a family member or friend accompanying the client? Did he or she have the same or different concerns as the client? If these were not formally addressed, give your assumptions.

_____

_____

_____

_____

Have you ever experienced problems swallowing (something getting stuck in your throat, liquids going down your trachea rather than your esophagus, choking)? What did you do to fix the problem? How did you feel during and after the incident?

_____

_____

_____

_____

◻ *Suggestions for Prediction*

Do you think you will be a clinician who enjoys helping people with dysphagia? What makes you think you will be either effective or ineffective with this category of client?

_____

_____

_____

_____

What types of disorders may have swallowing as a related problem? Think of both children and adults.

_____

_____

_____

_____

ANSWERS

A. The answers to Activity A are shown in **Table 4–2**.

Table 4–2 Swallowing Activity Answers

Goal: Client will independently use chin tuck before each swallow.
Verbal reminder: IIII
Visual reminder: III
Independent: I

C.

1. Thickening agent

2. Chin tuck

3. Tongue/lip strengthening exercises

4. Multiple swallow

CHAPTER 5

Language

THE FOCUS

The term *language* covers a lot of territory. It has been considered and examined in many different ways for the purpose of better understanding, describing, and treating difficulties an individual child or adult may experience with the communication message. We will briefly examine some of the ways language has been subdivided during assessment and/or treatment, but we begin with this caveat: no matter how you segment language, you *must* bring it back together into the whole and consider how the whole of language is impacting the communication process—the giving and receiving of information. To do this, it is crucial that language is examined and generalized to actual use across a variety of situations, partners, and levels of complexity.

Language has been subdivided in the following ways:

- *Expressive-receptive.* This is a very basic and broad segmentation. Terms such as *input* and *understanding* are synonymous with *receptive language*, while *output* and *production* are synonyms for *expressive language*. Language tests may assess receptive language components (assessed by client's pointing, selecting, or gesturing), expressive language components (assessed by client's verbalizing or signing), or both. When these discrete point assessment measures are utilized, many clinicians also will incorporate dynamic tasks and/or language sampling in the assessment to view expressive and receptive language as a whole.
- *Content-form-use.* Expressive and receptive language is further subdivided into areas of content or semantics, form or syntax/phonology/morphology, and use or pragmatics. Strengths and weaknesses of these interconnecting systems can help focus treatment sessions. We separate but remember to recombine.

- *Speaking-listening-reading-writing.* This separation reflects the mode of the message. Speaking (expressive)/listening (receptive) has been the traditional center of speech, language, and hearing treatment, but in the last 10 years, the literacy emphasis has broadened our scope of practice to increase the emphasis on writing (expressive)/reading (receptive). Especially in the preschool and school settings, all modes of language must be considered. A young child initially must learn the language, but as he/she grows, language becomes a critical tool for acquiring other learning.
- *Idiolect-dialect and accent-language.* Users of a language possess each of these components. The language or shared rule system such as English, Spanish, or sign language allows for communication with others who use the same language system. The dialects of a language are subsets of a language that reflect some rules that differ from the overriding language, yet not enough differences exist for them to be regarded as separate languages. Examples of dialects of English include Eastern American dialect, African American vernacular English, and Creole. Differences in the phonological or sound system of a dialect are referred to as accents. Foreign accents result from the speech characteristics of one language causing modifications in the phonological system when speaking another language. The idiolect reflects each individual's unique twists on his or her dialect. Individually created vocabulary and unique influences on pronunciation and inflections help fashion one's idiolect. During evaluation and treatment, SLPs should consider the idiolect and dialect when judging the accuracy of language use. It is essential to acknowledge that dialect differences, foreign accents, or isolated idiolectal modifications do not constitute a disorder, but rather a difference for which one may wish to enlist a speech therapist's help to modify.

THE ACTIVITY

A. Identify the first two components (expressive-receptive and content-form-use) that best fit the following 10 behaviors drawn from language objectives. Circle whether the example is a receptive or expressive task and then whether the primary focus is content, form, or use.

1. Repeat 10 new vocabulary words modeled during the book reading task.

expressive-receptive   content-form-use

2. Match the written verb with the picture referent.

expressive-receptive   content-form-use

3. Judge if the plural form of the word is correct or incorrect given an oral sentence.

      expressive-receptive   content-form-use

4. Give directions to locating an item in another room.

      expressive-receptive   content-form-use

5. Organize a grocery list by food category.

      expressive-receptive   content-form-use

6. Rewrite a sentence using the past tense.

      expressive-receptive   content-form-use

7. Initiate greetings.

      expressive-receptive   content-form-use

8. Write a check to pay the bill.

      expressive-receptive   content-form-use

9. Follow the direction from a recipe card with picture prompts.

      expressive-receptive   content-form-use

10. Choose between *right* and *left* when questioned in tasks throughout the school day.

      expressive-receptive   content-form-use

B. As a therapist, your role as a language model is important. To help foster developing into the best role model you can be, write a paragraph identifying your own language strengths and weaknesses and then transfer that information into the category summary chart (**Table 5–1**). For each weakness identify a self-remediation plan in the last column of the chart.

My language abilities …

_____

_____

_____

_____

Table 5–1 Observer Language Characteristics Summary Chart

Component	Description and Example of Strength(s)	Description and Example of Weakness(es)	Plan to Address Weakness(es) in Language
Expressive			
• Content			
• Form			
• Use			
Receptive			
• Content			
• Form			
• Use			
Speaking			
Listening			
Reading			
Writing			
Idiolect variations noted			
Dialect characteristics			
Language spoken			

AS YOU
OBSERVE... **C.** Write a paragraph to identify the strengths and weaknesses of the language therapist you are observing. Then transfer that information into **Table 5–2**. Note that the last column is to be used to record concrete examples of how the clinician addressed the categories in remediation.

The language clinician I am observing ...

_____

_____

_____

_____

AS YOU
OBSERVE... **D.** Write a paragraph identifying the strengths and weaknesses of the language client you are observing. Then transfer that information into **Table 5–3**. Note that the last column is to be used to plan how you would remediate the language weakness(es) in the sessions to come.

The language skills of the client I am observing ...

_____

_____

_____

_____

THE WRAP-UP

◻ *Suggestions for Reflections*

Which subdivision categories of language did you find most useful for self-evaluation, observed therapist evaluation, and client evaluation? Explain your answer.

_____

_____

_____

Table 5–2 Therapist Language Characteristics Summary Chart

Component	Description and Example of Strength(s)	Description and Example of Weakness(es)	Plan to Address Weakness(es) in Language
Expressive			
• Content			
• Form			
• Use			
Receptive			
• Content			
• Form			
• Use			
Speaking			
Listening			
Reading			
Writing			
Idiolect variations noted			
Dialect characteristics			
Language spoken			

Table 5–3 Client Language Characteristics Summary Chart

Component	Description and Example of Strength(s)	Description and Example of Weakness(es)	Plan to Address Weakness(es) in Language
Expressive			
• Content			
• Form			
• Use			
Receptive			
• Content			
• Form			
• Use			
Speaking			
Listening			
Reading			
Writing			
Idiolect variations noted			
Dialect characteristics			
Language spoken			

Explore your own idiolect. What is your language exposure history—what languages and dialects have you experienced? Which people have influenced your language—what were their dialects? Does your family or peer group have vocabulary or specific pronunciations that are part of your language? Name three words or pronunciations that are unique to you and a small circle of people you know. (Mine would be *kuchen*—a type of breakfast cake based on a German word, *hemplane*—a pronunciation for airplane that closes the open syllable at the beginning of the word based on a child's pronunciation error, and *fuzzel*—a family term for a piece of lint.)

_____

_____

_____

_____

◻ *Suggestions for Predictions*

If you plan a speech in your head, is this expressive language? Support your belief.

_____

_____

_____

_____

If you talk to yourself while alone in your car, is this expressive language? Support your belief.

_____

_____

_____

_____

If you read material that you cannot comprehend, is this receptive language? Support your belief.

_____

_____

_____

_____

Do you think the result of failing to bring the discrete components of language back to a whole would be too high or too low a representation of the client's language abilities? Support your answer.

_____

_____

_____

_____

What effect do you think *your* dialect will have on your obtaining a job and performing that job if you decide to practice speech, language, and hearing therapy in an area where most of the people speak a different dialect from the one you speak?

_____

_____

_____

_____

ANSWERS

A.

1. expressive and content

2. receptive and content

3. receptive and form

4. expressive and use

5. expressive and content

6. expressive and form

7. expressive and use

8. expressive and use

9. receptive and use

10. expressive and content

CHAPTER 6

Cognitive Therapy

THE FOCUS

The American Speech Language and Hearing Association developed nine areas in which students must show competency before beginning their clinical fellowship year. One of the nine areas deals with cognition. Cognition is how we process information as well as learn and remember information. People may experience problems with cognition as a result of a traumatic brain injury, stroke, or various other issues that manifest as problems with learning and remembering information. When speech-language pathologists work with cognition issues, they are conducting cognitive therapy or training. One type of cognitive training involves working on memory issues. When doing cognitive therapy, the clinician must make sure that the therapy activities are tied to functional goals. A functional goal is a measurable goal that increases a person's ability in his or her natural environment or in situations he or she encounters throughout his or her daily living routine.

Memory is one area of cognitive treatment. When working on memory issues, the clinician will need to gather information on the types of memory problems a person is experiencing and how those problems are affecting his life. For example, the clinician will need to know if the person is having problems with short-term memory, long-term memory, orientation to familiar places, or other types of difficulties. If a client is having a problem with short-term memory, the clinician may work on tasks to increase his ability in that particular area. The clinician may work on an activity such as reading a grocery list of five items and having the client repeat the list. If the client is successful with that number of items, the clinician should increase the number of items listed. If the client struggles with the list of five, the clinician may offer techniques such as chunking information to increase the number of items that can be remembered. For instance, if the grocery list contains the following items: grapes, cheese, bananas, milk, and bread, the clinician may teach the client to put similar foods together in her mind—perhaps something like this: grapes, bananas, bread, cheese, and milk, thus chunking the produce together and the dairy items together. By grouping similar items or making groupings of numbers, the client is learning the technique of chunking information.

Again, short-term memory is just one area of cognitive treatment. In most cases, when dealing with memory issues you will be working with or observing work with adult clients. There are rare instances when you may work with a child who is experiencing memory issues; however, most often you will see these problems in clients who have dementia, aphasia, traumatic brain injury, or some other problems that have occurred in the language center of the brain.

THE ACTIVITY

A. List ways in which the following items could be chunked:

1. Shirt, car, pants, shoes, keys

_____

_____

_____

_____

2. 525467342

_____

_____

_____

_____

3. Rocks, horses, elephants, trees, cats, flowers

_____

_____

_____

_____

4. Ocean, couch, mountains, table, chair, parks

_____

_____

_____

_____

B. Using context from the chapter, determine the definition of the following terms.

   1. Dementia:

_____

_____

_____

_____

   2. Aphasia:

_____

_____

_____

_____

   3. Traumatic brain injury:

_____

_____

_____

_____

   4. Chunking:

_____

_____

_____

_____

5. Functional goals:

_____

_____

_____

_____

6. Determine if the following scenarios are teaching memory techniques and explain why or why not.

Scenario 1. The clinician and client are looking through a magazine determining places to which the client would like to travel. The clinician asks the client why he/she is interested in traveling to these places.

_____

_____

_____

_____

Scenario 2. The clinician and client are looking through a magazine for recipes. They find a recipe the client indicates she would like to try. The clinician helps the client formulate a list of needed ingredients and cooking directions, asking the client to order the list of ingredients by similar items.

_____

_____

_____

_____

AS YOU OBSERVE... **C.** Think about the client you observed. Did the treatment session use any techniques to work on short-term memory? If so, list the technique and how that helps accomplish the goal. If not, develop a technique using some of the treatment materials that were used in the session.

_____

_____

_____

_____

THE WRAP-UP

◘ *Suggestions for Reflection*

Think about what you have observed with clients dealing with memory. Describe the treatment technique used with this client. Was this effective? Would you have tried something different? If so, what would you have tried?

_____

_____

_____

_____

What goals have been used with a client with memory problems? Were these goals considered functional? Why or why not? If not, how could you make them and the activities surrounding them functional?

_____

_____

_____

_____

◘ *Suggestions for Prediction*

What clients may have goals related to cognition? Determine some activities that you may use when working with these clients. Think about ways you may have to modify activities depending on their ability level.

_____

_____

_____

_____

How do you view yourself as a clinician working with clients with cognitive impairments? What are some questions you have about this population? Determine ways you could get answers for these questions (talking to supervisors, other clinicians, family members of the client). Write a functional goal related to a client with cognitive impairments; keep in mind what makes things functional for one client may not be functional for another.

_____

_____

_____

_____

ANSWERS

A.

1. Shirts, pants, shoes; keys, car

2. 525; 467; 342

3. Rocks, trees, flowers; horses, elephants, cats

4. Oceans, mountains, parks; couch, table, chair

B. Definitions:

1. *Dementia*: A progressive decline in cognitive function that is more significant than what is considered normal for that age.

2. *Aphasia*: Problems with expressing and understanding language.

3. *Traumatic brain injury*: Brain injury as a result of a sudden trauma.

4. *Chunking*: Putting information together in smaller pieces where the items relate to one another in a logical way to the user.

5. *Functional goals*: Goals that have meaning to the client's daily life.

C.

Scenario 1. The client and clinician are not working on memory issues; this is more a casual conversation where they may be working on vocabulary development but not directly working on memory.

Scenario 2. This is an example of working on short-term memory; by having the client using oral and written methods and having her put information in similar categories qualifies as using techniques to strengthen memory.

CHAPTER 7

Communication Modalities

THE FOCUS

Communicators utilize multiple modalities to give and receive messages. Think back to your last interaction before you began this observation. Did you speak, gesture with your hands, or change your expression or stance? Did you watch your partner while listening to the words spoken? When you wanted to get someone's attention across the room, did you first get eye contact, call out his or her name, or maybe even text message him or her? All communicators use multiple modalities. The communicators we are focusing on in this chapter are those learning to use or now using communication systems that rely more heavily on visual or tactile channels than verbal and auditory channels and include manual communication, assistive, and alternative technologies. We will refer to these individuals as using nontraditional communication modalities.

Consider this description of an imaginary girl who is severely compromised in both hearing and vision. While she was a baby, her parents used touch cues such as a pat on her hip to let her know they were going to lift her up. As a toddler she used object cues such as a lid from a sippy cup first as part of a receptive system to let her know a drink was coming and later as part of an expressive system to give to her mom to request a drink. Ultimately she became proficient in signing as her primary expressive means and tactile signing with her partner signing into her hands as her primary receptive means. She developed animated facial and body language which she used especially when outdoors. She occasionally gave a partner unfamiliar with sign language a written card asking him or her to print letters in her palm to facilitate communication. This story illustrates that communication systems are fluid and multidimensional because they must accommodate the individual's changing needs and abilities, the diversity of communication partners with a wide range of degree of familiarity with the speaker or the speaker's use of the modality, and the assortment of environments and situations in which the communication occurs. All three of these factors—the individual, the partner, and the environment—are relevant to all communicators but are even more important to consider for nontraditional modality users. All speakers are affected by factors such as fatigue and attention, but these may be even more critical to a nontraditional communication modality user, especially during the learning process. All speakers are affected by the skills of their communication partner, but this may be more evident when specialized training is needed to understand or respond to the message. All speakers need to modify their forms of providing communication depending on the environment but factors such as glare and environmental noise levels may be more detrimental to a nontraditional modality user.

The systems used to communicate are as heterogeneous and as unique and individual as the communicators who use them. No single diagnosis or label is associated with use of nontraditional communication modalities. Individuals who use nontraditional communication modalities include those with a number of different diagnoses including speech disorders, hearing loss, language disorders, cognitive delays, motor speech disorders, apraxia, autism, mutism, dysarthria, cerebral palsy, deafness, deafblindness, and many other diagnoses.

To illustrate this variety, the following examples of communication modalities users include a diagnosis, a specific use of a communication modality, and an indication of whether the example is of receptive or expressive use. These are written in person-first language to show our respect for the individual and the realization that the person is not defined by the disorder.

- An individual diagnosed with autism exchanging a picture for a desired item (expressive use).
- An individual diagnosed as deaf using sign language to discuss global warming with a colleague (expressive use).
- An individual diagnosed with cognitive delay using touch cues to be informed of his caregiver's plan to wash his face (receptive use).
- An individual diagnosed with cerebral palsy using an electronic communication device to participate in story time (expressive use).
- An individual diagnosed with apraxia using a letter board to signal the first letter of an unintelligible word (expressive use).
- An individual diagnosed as deafblind using tactile sign to receive the message of the commencement speaker (receptive use).

• An individual diagnosed with Down syndrome using sign language with his vocalization to request more of something (expressive use).

The list goes on and on.

THE ACTIVITY

A. Identify characteristics of communication modalities a clinician may have experienced by circling the term, or in some cases both terms, from each dichotomy presented below the example (expressive/receptive; verbal/nonverbal; technology involved/technology not involved).

1. Talking on the phone to new client.

> expressive/receptive;   verbal/nonverbal;
> technology involved/technology not involved

2. Watching a video of a session with the sound off.

> expressive/receptive;   verbal/nonverbal;
> technology involved/technology not involved

3. Completing an observational checklist while watching a therapy session through a viewing window.

> expressive/receptive;   verbal/nonverbal;
> technology involved/technology not involved

4. Having a conversation with a parent.

> expressive/receptive;   verbal/nonverbal;
> technology involved/technology not involved

5. Reading a clinic file.

> expressive/receptive;   verbal/nonverbal;
> technology involved/technology not involved

B. Find and circle the name of 10 disorders where communication modalities may be used in the word find puzzle in **Figure 7–1**.

Figure 7–1 **Word Find**

s	p	e	e	c	h	d	i	s	o	r	d	e	r
u	r	a	t	s	o	e	y	a	z	e	n	r	c
n	e	r	d	y	s	a	r	t	h	r	i	a	e
e	d	i	e	w	e	f	a	s	a	o	x	b	r
i	r	o	f	d	i	b	o	u	p	g	e	n	e
c	o	p	y	m	v	l	q	u	r	i	l	i	b
o	s	n	a	u	t	i	s	m	a	d	m	s	r
v	i	l	q	t	i	n	t	o	x	a	p		a
u	d	e	u	i	e	d	u	l	i	t	o	e	l
z	r	k	s	s	u	n	j	c	a	e	d	s	p
y	e	h	y	m	d	e	a	f	m	a	l	r	a
p	h	w	a	c	r	s	s	v	a	n	e	a	l
o	t	t	i	e	l	s	e	y	i	t	h	u	s
c	o	g	n	i	t	i	v	e	d	e	l	a	y

AS YOU OBSERVE...

C. Observe a speech, language, or hearing training session that has been identified as representing communication modalities. Answer the following classic *who, what, when, where,* and *why* focus questions.

1. Who is this client? Write a description of the individual. Identify or speculate on a probable diagnosis. Describe the individual's unique communication needs.

_____

_____

_____

_____

2. What is the communication modality system being taught or utilized? Describe both the receptive and expressive system in as much detail as possible. Also include a list of the modalities the *clinician* is using in this session.

_____

_____

_____

_____

3. When is the focus on the individual learning or using the communication modalities system? Describe how this system and the training provided are being individualized for this person.

_____

_____

_____

_____

4. Where is the awareness of the communication partner or environmental characteristics demonstrated? Describe such factors as the requirements to be a competent communication partner with this individual and how the material or communication device is positioned and accessed.

_____

_____

_____

_____

5. Why will this use of a nontraditional communication modality result in better communication interaction for this individual?

_____

_____

_____

_____

THE WRAP-UP

◻ *Suggestions for Reflections*

The classic questions sometimes include *how*. Ask and answer a how question concerning this observation.

_____

_____

_____

_____

Add the client you observed to the examples of communication modalities list at the end of the focus section. Include a diagnosis, a specific use of a communication modality, and an indication of whether the example is of receptive or expressive use.

_____

_____

_____

_____

Why is person-first language used?

_____

_____

_____

_____

Use your observation as a starting point to illustrate that communication modality systems are fluid and multidimensional.

_____

_____

_____

_____

☐ *Suggestions for Predictions*

What are the unique challenges of working in the area of communication modalities?

_____

_____

_____

_____

How have diagnostic labels changed over the years? (Hint: Consider the terms used to classify cognitive impairments or the changes in the terms associated with autism.) What factors influence diagnostic label changes?

_____

_____

_____

_____

ANSWERS

A.

1. expressive and receptive; verbal; technology involved

2. receptive; nonverbal; technology involved

3. expressive and receptive; verbal and nonverbal; technology involved

4. expressive and receptive; verbal and nonverbal; technology not involved

5. receptive; verbal; technology not involved

B. The word find answers are shown in **Figure 7–2**.

Figure 7–2 **Word Find Answers**

VERTICAL	HORIZONTAL
other disorder (bottom to top)	speech disorder
mutism	dysarthria
deafblindness	autism
apraxia	deaf
cerebral palsy	cognitive delay

s	p	e	e	c	h	d	i	s	o	r	d	e	r
	r										e		c
	e	d	y	s	a	r	t	h	r	i	a		e
	d										f	a	r
	r										b	p	e
	o		m								l	r	b
	s	a	u	t	i	s	m				i	a	r
	i		t								n	x	a
	d		i								d	i	l
	r		s								n	a	p
	e		m			d	e	a	f		e		a
	h										s		l
	t										s		s
c	o	g	n	i	t	i	v	e	d	e	l	a	y

CHAPTER 8

Social Aspects

THE FOCUS

What do challenging behaviors, ineffective social skills, and lack of communication opportunities have in common? Our answer to that question is, "use." Social aspects of communication are all about use! Whatever the client's communication system is, social aspects involve the pragmatics or use of that system to perform the communication functions desired. It is all about the use!

What population may experience difficulties with social aspects of communication? This can be a concern with any speech-language-hearing involved disorder and any age. However, deficits in the social use of communication are evident in persons with such varied diagnoses as autism spectrum disorder, traumatic brain injury, fetal alcohol syndrome, deafblindness, hearing disorders, and aphasia.

What would an example of social aspect remediation look like? Here is an anecdotal case of using a consultation-type approach to the social aspect issue. The family of a young child with a speech-language delay and challenging behaviors including tantruming and crying asked the clinician for suggestions on how to make going to the doctor a more manageable outing. She suggested that the family make a simple book to show the child what would happen at the doctor's office and what they expected of him and read it together several times before the scheduled appointment. The next day the family sent an e-mail attachment of a great looking e-book of a doctor's visit personalized with photos, names, and specific procedures that would occur. The family later reported positive outcomes and used the focused anticipation book technique for other potentially difficult communication situations such as the first day in a new preschool program. Clearly no one could customize situation-specific material better than the family. The clinician believed the factors of visual support provided by the pictures and text, clear articulation of positive behaviors (what he should do), clear explanation of the event (fewer unknowns), and visualization or pretend practice as possible reasons for the success this family experienced.

What training models have been used and evaluated that systematically address the needs of individuals with impairments in social aspects? Wankoff (2005) presents a description and an examination of the empirical evidence of a number of relevant approaches. Among the approaches described by Wankoff are applied behavior analysis (an intensive program using a stimulus–response reward sequence to target language or behavioral issues), TEACCH (Treatment and Education of Autistic and Related Communication-handicapped Children), a North Carolina statewide initiative that focuses on organized space and supports, and floor time model (an affect- and relationship-focused approach). Approaches that are frequently used in remediation of social skills include social stories, role playing, and peer modeling (to provide the individual use of replacement behaviors for inappropriate actions) and calendar systems and visual schedules to provide transparency and organization to the day or activity.

How might a clinician begin intervention for social aspects of communication? When working to decrease a challenging behavior, modify or replace ineffective social skills, or expand communication opportunities, a clinician first uses observational practices to identify patterns of behavior. Answering questions such as, "What happened before, during, and after the occurrence of the behavior? When, where, and with whom does the behavior frequently occur and just as importantly not occur? What communication function does this behavior seem to be expressing? And are there internal sensory or physical components that influence the occurrence of the behavior?" is a beginning step. Then the clinician joins with others from the client's remediation team, especially the family, and brainstorms probable reasons underlying the observed patterns. Next, the clinician looks to research literature, experience, and family input to develop an evidence-based plan and helps put that plan into action.

THE ACTIVITY

A. Pretend to be a part of the brainstorming team for the fictional child in the following scenario. Read the description of the behavior and answers to the observational questions. Then identify three possible reasons underlying the observed pattern and what in the scenario supports your reason. Compare your ideas with ours.

Scenario: Mary is a middle school student with significant cognitive, hearing, physical, and communication disorders. Her communication partners interpret her facial expressions, vocal inflections, and body postures as communicative messages. The challenging behavior that brought the team together is Mary's removal of her socks and shoes and kicking those around her during school. This behavior just began last week but is occurring daily.

The following are brief answers to the observational question:

What happened before, during, and after the occurrence of the behavior (shoe and sock removal and kicking)?

- Before—She pulls off her shoes and socks about 15 minutes after lunch each day.
- During—She is very persistent and keeps trying to remove the shoes even when the aide puts her hand over the shoes. Her body gets rigid and the loudness of her vocalizations increases. She continues thrashing and kicking until she is allowed to remove her shoes and socks. Mary is an easy-going child, so this is unusual behavior for her.
- After—After she removes her shoes and socks, she is calmer, appears to enjoy the attention she has been given, and is willing to put the shoes back on after about 50 minutes.

When, where, and with whom does the behavior frequently occur/ not occur?

Challenging behavior frequently occurs:

- When—After lunch.
- Where—On return to the classroom following lunch.
- With whom—Mary had a new aide in her class this week. It happened the first time with the new aide but later in the week with either aide or the teacher near her.

Challenging behavior infrequently occurs:

- When—The only time it did not occur this week was when the class went to the music room the period after lunch. The behavior did not occur when the group returned to the regular classroom.
- Where—Has not occurred in the music room.
- With whom—During music she was seated with a peer and university student buddy near the window. The new aide was not present.

What communication function does this behavior seem to be expressing?

- Escape—No.
- Protest—Only the thrashing and kicking seem to be protest for stopping her from removing her shoes and socks.

- Confusion—No.
- Others—Perhaps discomfort or need for assistance or attention.

Are there internal client sensory or physical components that influence the occurrence of the behavior?

- Auditory sensitivity—No
- Tactile sensitivity—Perhaps; shoes were closely examined to see if they were rubbing. A second pair of shoes was tried but the behavior remained.
- Headaches or other pain—Perhaps; parents were asked about change in medication but none had occurred. They reported Mary had experienced increased difficulty sleeping the last 2 weeks.
- Others—None.

Possible reason 1 underlying the observed pattern:

_____

Explanation:

_____

_____

_____

_____

Possible reason 2 underlying the observed pattern:

_____

Explanation:

_____

_____

_____

_____

Possible reason 3 underlying the observed pattern:

_____

Explanation:

_____

_____

_____

_____

Possible reason 4 underlying the observed pattern:

_____

Explanation:

_____

_____

_____

_____

AS YOU OBSERVE…

B. Identify a specific challenging behavior or a specific ineffective social skill of the child you are observing. Do your best to answer the observational questions below. Write a paragraph describing the behavior, possible cause, and the intervention plan the clinician is following.

Answer the following questions examining the behavior you selected:

What happened before, during, and after the occurrence of the behavior?

- Before

_____

_____

- During

_____

_____

- After

_____

_____

When, where, and with whom does the behavior frequently occur/not occur?

Challenging behavior frequently occurs:

- When

  _____

  _____

- Where

  _____

  _____

- With whom

  _____

  _____

Challenging behavior infrequently occurs:

- When

  _____

  _____

- Where

  _____

  _____

- With whom

  _____

  _____

What communication function does this behavior seem to be expressing?

- Escape

  _____

  _____

- Protest

  _____

  _____

• Confusion

_____

_____

• Others

_____

_____

Are there internal client sensory or physical components that influence the occurrence of the behavior?

• Auditory sensitivity

_____

_____

• Tactile sensitivity

_____

_____

• Headaches or other pain

_____

_____

• Others

_____

_____

Paragraph describing the behavior, possible causes, and therapy observed:

_____

_____

_____

_____

THE WRAP-UP

◻ *Suggestions for Reflection*

Did you have access to as much information on the behavior you described as the authors did about Mary? What other key information would you like to know about your client's behavior?

_____

_____

_____

_____

How would the therapy plan differ if the reason underlying Mary's behavior is being too hot vs. seeking attention/interaction?

_____

_____

_____

_____

How would you modify the list of observational questions? What questions would you add, delete, and/or modify?

_____

_____

_____

_____

Write a definition of challenging behaviors in your own words.

_____

_____

_____

_____

◻ *Suggestions for Predictions*

If we had asked, what do basketball, football, and baseball have in common, you might have said "ball." While "ball" is a dandy answer, it is surely not the only answer. "Team sport," "athletics," or "involves coaches" would have been fine, too. Go back to our opening paragraph concerning the commonality of challenging behaviors, ineffective social skills, and lack of communication opportunities and provide another answer instead of "use" and your reasoning for the choice.

_____

_____

_____

_____

What three key words would you use when doing a library or internet search for therapy approaches for a client with a deficit in social aspects of communication?

_____

_____

_____

_____

ANSWERS

A.

Possible reason 1 underlying the observed pattern: Mary is too hot after lunch, perhaps due to some changes in her body's systems.

Why? The taking off shoes and socks would make her cooler. The music room seating by the window might have been cooler so music class was fine. The increased sleeping disturbance could be reflecting changes in her body's systems.

Possible reason 2 underlying the observed pattern: Mary wanted the attention/interaction of the new aide.

Why? The change corresponded to introduction of the new person. The aide was not present at music and Mary had the attention of a peer and university buddy.

Possible reason 3 underlying the observed pattern: Mary is tired after lunch and sees taking off her shoes and socks as the first step toward a nap.

Why? She is sleeping badly, so being tired is likely. The removal of footwear could be part of her napping routine.

Possible reason 4 underlying the observed pattern: Mary has developed a food allergy.

Why? The discomfort seemed to happen after lunch. While we noted lunch as a before-the-behavior factor, we did not look specifically at what was consumed differently on the music day.

REFERENCE

Wankoff, L. S. (2005). *Innovative methods in language intervention: Treatment outcome measures. Can the data support the claims?* Austin, TX: pro-ed.

CHAPTER 9

Hearing

THE FACTS

One aspect of an audiologist's job is to evaluate hearing. The results are plotted on an audiogram in order to interpret the type and severity of hearing loss for each ear. Tympanometry is a test that looks at the function of the tympanogram and middle ear. This test gives information such as whether the client has fluid or some other outer or middle ear problem. For the hearing test various frequencies (or pitches) are tested from a low frequency (250 Hz) to a high frequency (8000 Hz). The audiologist will obtain the client's threshold at each of the frequencies tested. Threshold is the softest sound a person can hear. You will notice that the audiologist does not document each response from the client on the audiogram; instead he or she documents only the softest sound the person consistently hears or the threshold for each pitch tested.

There are ranges of hearing loss from normal hearing (0–15 dB Hearing Level) to profound (90+ dB HL). After the audiologist obtains thresholds at the various frequencies and plots the thresholds for each, you may observe him testing the client's ability to understand words. The first test is known as a speech reception threshold and looks at the softest level at which the person can understand speech stimuli. The next test you may observe is a speech discrimination test. During this test, the audiologist is trying to determine how well the person can understand speech in an optimal environment (i.e., at a comfortable loudness level for the client, in quiet). The results of the tests should all match; the speech reception threshold should be around the same level as the thresholds for the speech frequencies, and the client should be able to understand a fair amount of the words when they are presented in optimal conditions. If the test results do not align, the audiologist will need to do further assessments to determine the origin of the problem.

On the audiogram report shown in **Figure 9–1**, you will notice that the numbers on the *x* axis are frequency (pitch) from 250 Hz to 8000 Hz. On the *y* axis, you will notice the numbers are an indication of decibels (loudness) with soft sounds at the top of the graph and loud sounds at the bottom of the graph. Notice the ranges of hearing; for example, 41–55 dB is in the moderate hearing loss range.

A case history is extremely important before testing a client. The audiologist can gain vital information from the case history, which can help her determine what tests are important and if she needs to be looking for something specific. An example of this would be if a child came in with delayed speech and language. The audiologist would want to know if the child was given and passed a hearing screening at birth, if he has a history of ear infections, if there is any family history of hearing loss, or if there were any problems with the pregnancy or birth. Another example would be an adult who was having decreased hearing and dizziness. The audiologist would want to know how long the person had been experiencing this, if the symptoms have ever occurred before, if there have been any recent incidents of head trauma or other medical condition, and if the person is taking any medications, and if so what they are and how long the patient has been taking them.

If you are interested in becoming a speech-language pathologist, you may not go through a rotation in your clinical practicum sites that includes audiologic evaluations where thresholds are obtained; however, you will be required to show competency with hearing screenings. The difference between finding thresholds and completing screenings is that with screenings, there is no interpretation of the information. Screenings are pass/fail only. Various frequencies are tested, but the audiometer (equipment that is used to test hearing) is set at a particular level for each frequency and the client either hears the tone or does not. If the client does not hear the tone at the set frequency, it is considered a fail. You will need to check with your supervisor to determine the protocol for failed hearing screenings. It is important to note if you are asked to do hearing screenings at your work site, you will need to make sure that you have an audiometer and that the piece of equipment is calibrated annually. When screening hearing, you will need to make sure that the room in which you are screening hearing is quiet enough that nothing will alter the validity of the test. In some cases, you may be asked to screen hearing in the cafeteria or other area that may not be very quiet; make sure to advocate for yourself and your clients and request a quieter room.

Hearing is vital to speech-language development. When children have a hearing loss, even a mild hearing loss, they do not pick up on all the nuances of language. For instance, children who hear in the normal range tend to pick up things such as rhythm and prosody of language just by being exposed to someone else's conversation. A child with even a mild hearing loss may not pick up on these things by overhearing it because she has to be focused on that conversation before she would really notice those things. Another example would be a child with a high-frequency hearing loss. This

Western Carolina University
Speech and Hearing Clinic
G30 McKee Building
Cullowhee, NC 28723
(828) 227-7251
(828) 227-7457

NAME: _____

DATE OF BIRTH: _____

DATE OF TEST: _____

PURE TONE AUDIOMETRY (RE: ANSI 1996)

OTOSCOPY: _____

KEY		
LEFT	STIMULUS	RIGHT
X	AIR	o
□	AIR MASK	Δ
>	BONE	<
]	BONE MASK	[
↘	NO RESPONSE	↙
SOUND FIELD - S		
AIDED SOUND FIELD - A		

TYMPANOMETRY (226 Hz/1000Hz)

EAR	LEFT	RIGHT
EAR CANAL VOLUME Cm³		

TEST TYPE
STANDARD
PLAY
CDR/VRA
BOA

TRANSDUCER
INSERT
CIRCUMAURAL
SOUND FIELD

RELIABILITY
EXCELLENT
GOOD
FAIR
POOR

TYMPANOMETER _____

SPEECH AUDIOMETRY

	PTA	SRT/SAT	Speech Recognition	Speech Recognition	MCL	UCL
Right			%	%		
Masking						
Left			%	%		
Masking						
SOUND FIELD			%	%		
RIGHT AIDED			%	%		
LEFT AIDED			%	%		
BINAURAL			%	%		

AUDIOMETER _____

OTOACOUSTIC EMISSIONS (OAEs)

EMISSION TYPE USED	TEST TYPE PERFORMED
Transient	OAE complete
Distortion product	OAE screening

OAE results:
Right ear
Left ear

OAE unit _____

HEARING AID INFORMATION
RIGHT AID: _____
LEFT AID: _____

HISTORY/IMPRESSIONS/RECOMMENDATIONS: _____

AUDIOLOGIST: _____

Figure 9–1 Audiogram

child may miss final consonants because at the end of words and sentences, speakers typically lose volume, and unless it is quiet and the child is paying attention to facial cues, he may miss the final sounds of words. Have you ever been exposed to loud noise, such as at a concert, and when you leave your ears feel full—almost as if you are not hearing very well; or perhaps you have had a cold and your ears feel stopped up and it seems you are struggling to hear? Perhaps you noticed during those times that it was difficult to hear certain speech sounds, particularly in the presence of background noise. Now imagine that you hear like that all the time and that you are just learning a new language. Think of all the problems you may experience learning some of the words, sounds, or even the rhythm of that language. Hearing loss can make it very difficult to learn certain aspects of a language, and if a child is just learning how to talk and interact with others, she will likely have some speech and language delays. For this reason, early detection and intervention are very important. Luckily, most states implement newborn hearing screenings, meaning the babies have a hearing test before they leave the hospital. This has helped make sure children with hearing difficulties are identified early in life. As speech-language pathologists and audiologists, you will likely be faced with clients with hearing loss. It is important to know the implications of hearing loss and learn how you can best assist those clients with their speech and language.

THE ACTIVITY

A. Circle T for true and F for false. For false answers, write a true statement.

1. T / F A client's threshold is documented on an audiogram.

_____

_____

2. T / F Frequency is a measurement of the level of loudness the person needs for the tone to be heard.

_____

_____

3. T / F A simple case history consisting of the person's name and demographic information is all that is needed prior to testing.

_____

_____

4. T / F A screening is pass/fail only.

_____

_____

5. T / F Performing a hearing screening is within the scope of practice for an SLP.

_____

_____

B. It is important for an SLP to be able to read the information on an audiogram. Using the audiogram in **Figure 9–1** (including information from the key) and information in this chapter, answer the following questions and explain why this is important information for an SLP:

   1. List the severity ranges for hearing.

_____

_____

   2. This is important because ...

_____

_____

_____

_____

   3. What symbols are used for the right and left ears when testing using air conduction?

_____

_____

   4. This is important because ...

_____

_____

_____

_____

   5. How is threshold documented?

_____

_____

6. This is important because ...

_____

_____

_____

_____

THE WRAP-UP

◻ *Suggestions for Reflection*

Think about the client you just observed. Describe what information was obtained from the case history that let the audiologist know what problems the client was experiencing.

_____

_____

_____

_____

Explain how the test results matched (how did the speech testing go along with the thresholds; were there any significant problems understanding speech signals?).

_____

_____

_____

_____

◻ *Suggestions for Predictions*

Why do you think people are reluctant to have hearing evaluations? What information could be given to people to make them feel more comfortable?

_____

_____

_____

_____

Think of a time when you have had problems hearing or when you have been communicating with someone who seems to have problems hearing. If you or that person were going to have a hearing evaluation, what information would be helpful to include on a case history form?

_____

_____

_____

_____

ANSWERS

A.

    1. True.

    2. False—Frequency is the specific pitch of tone being tested.

    3. False—A thorough case history is vital before beginning testing.

    4. True.

    5. True.

B.

    1. 0–15 dB—Normal hearing sensitivity; 16–25 dB—Slight hearing loss; 26–40 dB—Mild hearing loss; 41–55 dB—Moderate hearing loss; 56–70 dB—Moderately severe hearing loss; 71–90 dB—Severe hearing loss; 91+ dB—Profound hearing loss.

    2. This is important to know because a person will typically have more difficulty communicating the greater the hearing loss, and knowing the ranges helps explain how a person could have various hearing thresholds that are different but within the same range of hearing loss.

    3. Right ear air conduction—O, left ear air conduction—X.

    4. This is important because knowing the symbols will allow you to read audiograms from various sources.

    5. Threshold is documented by the correct symbol being noted one time only at the softest sound the person can consistently hear at a particular frequency.

    6. This is important because each frequency should have only one documented symbol for each ear for air conduction and then bone conduction. Again, this helps a person to be able to read audiograms from various sources and in clinic-to-clinic and longevity comparisons.

Supplemental Areas

CHAPTER 10

Intelligibility

THE FOCUS

A core concept in the correction of sound disorders is intelligibility or how well the client can be understood when speaking. Intelligibility is often estimated and provided as a percentage of time the individual is understood by the listener. This subjective measure is affected by how well the listener knows the individual and the context of the message being given. Think about playing charades or a word guessing game. The better the communicating players know each other (e.g., family vs. strangers) and the more precise context of the message (e.g., category of clue vs. any possible word), the easier it is for the listening partner to guess the message. Often intelligibility is specified as percentage understood by a familiar listener or by an unfamiliar listener. Sometimes, actual numbers of words are counted and the percentage is calculated by dividing the number of words understood by the total number of words spoken, and then this result is multiplied by 100 (Shipley & McAfee, 1998). Both the estimated and calculated measures of intelligibility provide useful pre-post measures of articulation skill. Remember that intelligibility improves as children develop their sound systems. When children begin to speak, their intelligibility scores are low especially to unfamiliar listeners but by the time they reach 5 years of age, most are highly intelligible, even to unfamiliar listeners.

Because intelligibility is developmental, it is important that a clinician can determine a client's age in years and months when given a date of birth. To calculate an age, take today's date arranged in order of year, month, day, and subtract from that the client's birthday also in the year, month, day order. Remember that this is not your typical base-10 subtraction problem. When you borrow 1 from the years column, you carry 12 months and when you borrow 1 from the months column you carry 30 days. As a final step, if the days column results are 15 or over, then add 1 to the months total, and if the days column result is under 15, then make no change to the months total. If today's date were January 10, 2009, and the client was born on November 20, 2005, you would set the problem up as follows:

date	year	month	day		year	month	day
today	2009	1	10	after borrowing,	2008	12	40
birthday	−2005	11	20	restated as	−2005	11	20
					3	1	20

Age = 3 years, 2 months

THE ACTIVITY

A. Practice determining the estimated and calculated intelligibility scoring for the phonetically transcribed sample provided in No. 1. Then practice determining age given a client's birthday for the three examples provided. After you have completed your calculations of intelligibility and age, check the answer key for comparison.

1. Use the sample below to make intelligibility judgments. Read the sample written phonetically and estimate the intelligibility. Next complete the calculations (note (—) in place of the word means the word was not understood):

/ /maɪ (—) lɪv baɪ (—) // in aur twi // (—) (—) fit // wɪl ju (—) gɪv mi (—) aɪs krim koun//

First reading record of the intelligibility estimate = _____ percent

Calculated intelligibility = ___ correct words/ ___ total words × 100 = _____ percent

2. Calculate the age of the following three people using a different "today's date" (provided) for each person.

Person A was born on March 9, 1952; for purpose of this activity, today's date is April 10, 2010. Client A is _____ years, _____ months old.

Person B born on January 30, 1999; for purpose of this activity, today's date is January 3, 2009. Client B is _____ years, _____ months old.

Person C born on October 9, 2001; for purpose of this example today's date is September 25, 2010. Client C is _____ years, _____ months old.

AS YOU OBSERVE...

B. Listen to the session of a child or adult with sound errors you are observing for about 5–10 minutes. From that brief sample, estimate the percentage of intelligibility and record your estimate and whether you would be considered a familiar or unfamiliar listener. Now select a time when the client is engaged in a conversation or a monologue (not drill work) and use pluses (+) and minuses (–) to represent each word the client articulates. Follow the formula to determine the intelligibility. The longer and more conversational the sample you use, the more accurately your measure should reflect the client's understandability. The primary reason for completing this activity is to center your attention on the speech production of the articulation client you are observing.

  1. Record of intelligibility determination

   a. Intelligibility estimate

   Time of observation = _____ minutes.

   Activity observed = _____.

   Estimate of intelligibility = _____ percent by _____ (familiar or unfamiliar) listener.

   b. Calculated intelligibility

   Time of observation = _____ minutes.

   Activity observed = _____.

   Number of words understood (marked as +) = _____

   Number of words not understood (marked as –) =_____

   Total number of words (No. + and No. –) = _____

   Calculated intelligibility = _____ (No. +) / _____ (No. + and No. –) × 100 = _____

   by _____ (familiar or unfamiliar) listener.

THE WRAP-UP

☐ Suggestions for Reflection

How close were your estimated and calculated figures? Support one of these measures as being the most accurate.

_____

_____

_____

_____

What factors contribute to your rating of intelligibility? Familiarity of listener and amount of contextual information present (shared or unshared experiences) were identified as two factors that influence intelligibility. Think of other factors that influence how easy it is to understand a speaker.

_____

_____

_____

_____

◘ *Suggestions for Predictions*

Intelligibility scoring is influenced by the familiarity of the listener. In what other ways does familiarity or knowledge of the client influence the therapeutic process?

_____

_____

_____

_____

Is it easier to plan for a new client or one whom you have seen for many months?

_____

_____

_____

_____

Is it possible that knowing a client for a length of time can be a negative factor?

_____

_____

_____

_____

Write the instructions for determining age when given a date of birth. Name two reasons this is important to an SLP.

_____

_____

_____

_____

ANSWERS

A.

1. / /maɪ (—) lɪv baɪ (—) // in aur twi // (—) (—) fit // wɪl ju (—) gɪv mi (-) aɪs krim koun//

Translation: My ___ live by ___. In our tree. ___ ___ feet. Will you ___ give me ___ ice cream cone?

Estimate of intelligibility was probably about 50 percent; calculated intelligibility score was 14 words understood/20 possible words × 100 = 70 percent.

2. Person A

date	year	month	day		year	month	day
today	2010	4	10	or restated	2010	4	10
birthday	−1952	3	9	as	−1952	3	9
					58	1	1

Person A is 58 years, 1 month old.

Person B

date	year	month	day		year	month	day
today	2009	1	3	restated as	2008	12	33
birthday	−1999	1	30		−1999	1	30
					9	11	3

Person B is 9 years, 11 months old.

Person C

date	year	month	day		year	month	day
today	2010	9	25	or restated	2009	21	25
birthday	−2001	10	9	as	−2001	10	9
					8	11	16

Person C is 9 years old.

REFERENCE

Shipley, K. G., and McAfee, J. G. (1998). *Assessment in speech-language pathology: A resource manual* (2nd ed.). San Diego, CA: Singular.

CHAPTER 11

Sign Language

THE FOCUS

Almost everyone is aware of the use of sign language as a mode of communication for persons who are deaf or hard of hearing. The use of manual communication with the normal hearing population has increased over the past decade. Many parents use sign language to help their infants develop more specific communication techniques in order to allow their children to request items such as food, drink, or more long before their speech is developed enough to request them verbally. Sign language may also be used in therapy for children who are becoming increasingly frustrated with speech, who do not have the abilities needed for verbal communication, or who need a temporary system until they are able to use a verbal mode.

There are cases in which children become so frustrated by their difficulty with verbal communication that behavior issues occur. Imagine a child who has phonological problems. Phonological problems are consistent sound errors such as fronting (when the child says all back sounds as front sounds), initial or final consonant deletion, or stopping (when sounds such as fricatives become stops). Most children with phonological problems are difficult to understand. The child is using speech and language in a way that he believes is correct, but most people are not able to understand him. Adults may ask the child to repeat himself several times and still not be able to understand. In this case, the child may become frustrated and refuse to talk. Teaching this child with phonological problems some signs may help alleviate some of the frustration while he is working on his sound system.

Another case of frustration could occur with an apraxic client, especially a child. By teaching a child (or adult if needed) some other forms of communication in order to have her wants and needs met and reduce some of the anxiety, you as the clinician may help to facilitate her verbal communication by reducing some of the pressures associated with speaking. Most of the time, adults have found other forms of communication, such as writing, but children may need an alternative method of communicating to get their needs met. Sign language can serve as that alternative method as some basic signs can be helpful for all those involved with the child, and the family does not have to carry any additional equipment (such as augmentative and alternative communication devices) in order to communicate.

In the past, there were some concerns about teaching a child sign language, in that people were afraid the child would rely solely on sign language and not use his verbal communication. Evidence has shown that use of sign is not a detriment to a child learning to speak. It is important to keep in mind that you always couple the signs with words. When you are teaching the signs you teach them along with the word the sign represents. So if you are teaching the sign for food, you also say the word *food* simultaneously. In therapy, you want to always couple signs with words and teach the parents and children the importance of using signs with words and always encouraging the child to verbalize as they are signing. Frequently used signs are included in this chapter. For the child dealing with phonological processes, his or her speech may not be clear, but the sign language will reinforce the words he or she is using, and the child can have his or her needs met with a reduced level of frustration. Keep in mind you want to expand the communication skills so if the child signs "more" and approximates a word for *more*, you as the clinician want to provide a good language model and say something like, "You want more" or "I want more."

Manual communication can provide your clients and their families options for increased communication with decreased frustration. Always include the family in the selection of the signs and teach the family members the use of sign with verbal communication. There are resources available such as books and posters that provide easy-to-understand visual images for learning various signs.

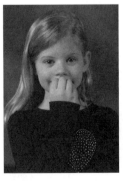   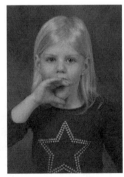

Figure 11–1 Eat   **Figure 11–2 Drink**

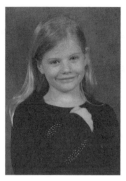

Figure 11–3 **Please**

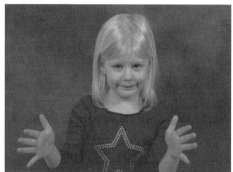

Figure 11–4 **Finished**

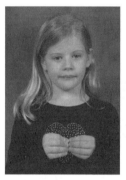

Figure 11–5 **More**

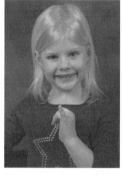

Figure 11–6 **I**

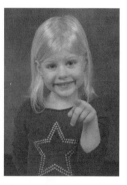

Figure 11–7 **You**

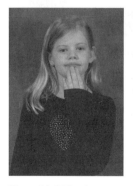

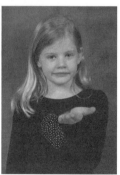

Figure 11–8 **Thank you**

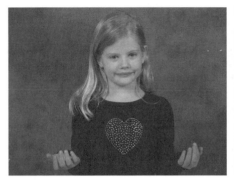

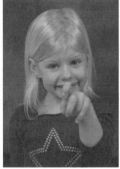

Figure 11–9 **Want**   Figure 11–10 **Need**

THE ACTIVITY

A. Label the following signs.

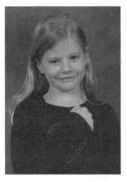
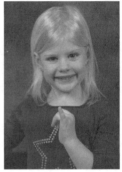
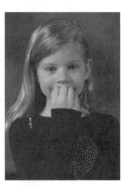

1. _____   2. _____   3. _____

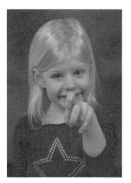 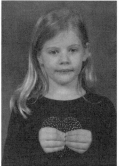

4. _____   5. _____

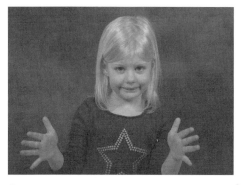

6. _____

G. Think about the client you just observed. What signs would be help-ful to the client, his or her family, or the clinician to decrease frustra-tion and communicate more effectively?

_____

_____

_____

_____

THE WRAP-UP

◻ *Suggestions for Reflection*

Why do you think people at one time were reluctant to teach sign to babies and toddlers with normal hearing?

_____

_____

_____

_____

How could you use sign language to increase the length of utterance for children or adults?

_____

_____

_____

_____

◻ *Suggestions for Predictions*

What are some disorders that were not listed in the chapter for which sign language could be beneficial with teaching?

_____

_____

_____

_____

How do you talk to a parent about introducing some signs when he has a huge concern that his child will never be verbal and he has been reluctant about implementing signs or any other communication device?

_____

_____

_____

_____

ANSWERS

A.

    1. Please

    2. I

    3. Eat

    4. Need

    5. More

    6. Finished

CHAPTER 12

Augmentative and Alternative Communication (AAC)

THE FOCUS

What can be done to assist a person who cannot communicate using his voice? Augmentative and alternative communication (AAC) may be the answer. There are several levels to AAC, including unaided AAC and aided AAC. Within the aided AAC category, there are two levels (low-tech and high-tech devices). For each client using AAC, it must be determined what level will work best for that individual and his lifestyle.

Unaided AAC does not require any outside or external device. The options may include manual communication, facial gestures, body posture, and vocalizations. The benefits to using unaided AAC are that the client does not have to rely on anything external and will not have to keep up with a device. Gestures and facial expressions are typically understood by almost everyone, thus allowing some communication between many different partners. Some disadvantages of unaided AAC are the client must have control of gross motor movements and facial expressions, the amount of communication may be limited, and the time required to communicate may be expanded depending on how well the communication partners understand the gestures, vocalizations, or signs.

An external device is used when aided AAC is chosen as the mode of communication. Devices may not require batteries or electricity (low-tech devices) or may implement electronics in order to store and retrieve messages (high-tech devices). Examples of low-tech devices include picture exchange boards and paper and pen. There are various companies that make high-tech devices that have a voice output, and when the client selects an image, the device will say the word that is programmed into the device. High-tech devices vary in size, weight, and the amount of information they store. Devices have different options as to how the message is chosen. For instance, the client may be able to touch the object using a finger or pointing device, or the device might be programmed to respond to eye movements.

In many states, there are government-supported programs or centers that have various types of equipment for loaning out to clinicians and/or families. These centers make it possible to see what type of device works best for the client and his or her family. Many insurance companies will cover the cost of the device after it has been determined that the client can be successful with the device. Because the devices can be costly, the clinician will want to make sure they know what resources are available in the state and community and know the requirements of the insurance company if the client is going to submit a claim for reimbursement. The clinician must also be cognizant of possible modifications available for the device to reflect changes in the client's skills and needs. Some schools have devices available for the students. If the device belongs to the school, there are likely rules about the student being allowed to take the device home or to work sites or field trips. Because the client will be more successful when she has the same equipment available to her throughout her entire day, the clinician may need to assist clients/families in obtaining devices through other sources.

In therapy, you may observe the clinician working with the client to learn to communicate effectively using the AAC device. For instance, if the client is just being acclimated to the device, you may see the clinician using a closed-set task where the client has a limited number of choices and the clinician will have the client answer a question or have the client request something using one of the two choices. When the client is successful with only a couple of choices, the clinician may introduce more choices or ask open-ended questions so the client can increase his or her options.

If you are observing clients who have been using their AAC device for some time, you may have the chance to observe the clinician and a client reprogramming a device to better meet the client's needs or engaging in true conversational interactions. An example of this may be with a client who has had a stroke and has intact cognitive skills but lacks the ability to say the words he intends to say due to a breakdown in the brain's signal to the articulators. Such a client may be extremely successful using an AAC device, but he may find he needs to reprogram the device to use different words or symbols in order to meet his everyday communicative needs. In some cases, a family member may learn to reprogram the device, but in others the client would return to the SLP or teacher in order to have the device reprogrammed and to make sure the device is functional for him. Making sure a team approach is used and the client is using the same device across settings is vital for success with AAC. If clients have to change devices in different settings, it makes it very hard for them to really learn one system and be able to use it effectively. When deciding on the AAC device to use with a client, the clinician must take this into consideration.

THE ACTIVITY

A. Consider the factors of technology and equipment by completing the items below.

    1. What is the difference between a low-tech and a high-tech AAC device?

_____

_____

_____

_____

    2. What is the difference between aided and unaided AAC?

_____

_____

_____

_____

B. Rate the following AAC devices as (1) low-tech or high-tech and (2) aided or unaided by circling the correct terms after each device example. Then draw and label a sketch of an example of each device to demonstrate your knowledge (stick figures are fine).

    1. Signaling button—a device that has a button that is pressed in order to make a selection. The most basic one has a single large button similar to that shown in the Easy Button commercials. To what is the signaling button attached?

        low-tech/high-tech   *aided/unaided*

SKETCH

2. Paper and pen

low-tech/high-tech   *aided/unaided*

SKETCH

3. Sign-language

low-tech/high-tech   *aided/unaided*

SKETCH

4. Computerized system that produces a ticker-tape-type readout

low-tech/high-tech   *aided/unaided*

SKETCH

5. Voice output device

low-tech/high-tech   *aided/unaided*

SKETCH

6. Gestures

low-tech/high-tech   *aided/unaided*

SKETCH

7. Alphabet board to indicate the letters not clear to the listener or to spell out the message

low-tech/high-tech   *aided/unaided*

SKETCH

8. Symbol book of picture choices an individual commonly uses

low-tech/high-tech   *aided/unaided*

SKETCH

9. Eye gaze Plexiglas board to visually select between spaced picture or word choices

low-tech/high-tech   *aided/unaided*

SKETCH

10. Electrolarynx to provide the sound source when the larynx has been removed

low-tech/high-tech   *aided/unaided*

SKETCH

C. Answer these questions about the session you just observed. Draw and label a detailed sketch of the client using his/her AAC device.

1. What type AAC device was used? Please be as specific as possible. Include name and descriptive characteristics for high-tech devices and size, materials, and symbols used for low-tech devices.

_____

_____

_____

_____

2. At what stage was the client with regard to using his or her device?

_____

_____

_____

_____

3. What is the goal you believe was being addressed for this client with this device?

_____

_____

_____

_____

4. What are two ways this device could be modified in the future to reflect changes in the client's skill level or communication circumstances?

_____

_____

_____

_____

SKETCH

THE WRAP-UP

◻ *Suggestions for Reflection*

What factors determine what type of device is chosen for a client?

_____

_____

_____

_____

How would the goals differ for a client just learning to use a device versus a client who has been using the same device (with success) for an extended period of time?

_____

_____

_____

_____

Is there a center in your community for obtaining AAC equipment? Identify the name, address, and phone number of the center closest to your anticipated work site. What types of equipment are available? Is the equipment available for check-out to families, clinicians, or both? What are the center's policies for checking out devices?

_____

_____

_____

_____

☐ *Suggestions for Predictions*

How will you assist a client to learn to use a device in various settings (not just the clinic setting)? What are some factors that might change the level of difficulty for a client between the clinic setting and his or her everyday life?

_____

_____

_____

_____

How could you as the clinician aid a child who is learning to use an AAC device in her regular classroom? How could you incorporate other students in this learning process?

_____

_____

_____

_____

Why is it essential that a team of involved individuals participate in AAC selection, training, and use? Write a scenario about an individual in need of an AAC device. Provide age, reason for AAC need, relevant strengths and limitations of the client, situations in which he needs to communicate, and anticipated partners. Name five people who should be on the AAC assessment/treatment team:

_____

_____

_____

_____

ANSWERS

A.

1. A low-tech device requires no battery or electricity whereas a high-tech device is a device that requires some type of power source.

   2. An unaided AAC device does not require any external equipment, whereas an aided device requires something external to the client.

B. Your sketches should resemble the figures below.

   1. High-tech/aided

   2. Low-tech/aided

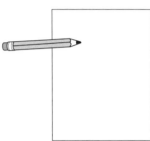

   3. Low-tech/unaided

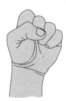

   4. High-tech/aided

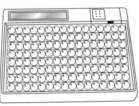

   5. High-tech/aided

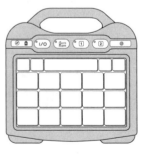

6. Low-tech/unaided

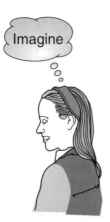

7. Low-tech/aided

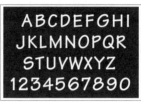

8. Low-tech/aided

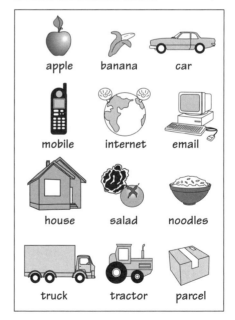

9. Low-tech/aided

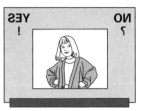

10. High-tech/aided

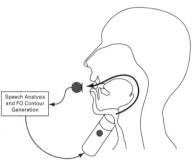

CHAPTER 13

Hearing Aids

Hearing aids are the most common form of amplification recommended by audiologists. There are other types of amplification, such as assistive listening devices, cochlear implants, and implantable amplification; however, as either an audiologist or speech-language pathologist, chances are you will be working with clients who have hearing aids more often than any other amplification device. Because of this, it is important to understand that hearing aids come in all shapes and sizes with various features. Audiologists will make the recommendation for the hearing aid and perform the fitting and orientation to the hearing aid, but speech-language pathologists will often be asked to troubleshoot problems or assist a client with a hearing aid. This chapter will provide a brief overview of the major components of hearing aids and some basic types and styles.

All hearing aids have a microphone (where the sound enters), a processor (some type of strategy the hearing aid uses to transfer the acoustic signal to an electric signal that it can process and adjust), an amplifier (what increases the level of the sound), a receiver (the component that transfers the electrical signal back to an acoustic signal and sends the signal to the ear), and a power source (battery). Most hearing aids use digital processing technology. Using digital processing allows the signal to undergo various modifications (increasing loudness, compressing the large number of frequencies to a smaller frequency range, transposing the higher frequencies to lower frequencies) while keeping the signal as clear as possible. Digital hearing aids also optimize the battery life. Hearing aid batteries are very small and typically last between 10 and 14 days, depending on the amount of time the hearing aids are on every day.

Hearing aids come in many different sizes. Behind-the-ear (also known as BTE) hearing aids have an ear mold that is inserted in the ear and is coupled to the hearing aid. In-the-ear (ITE) hearing aids fill the entire concha bowl of the ear. In-the-canal (ITC) hearing aids fit in the canal so the opening to the external auditory meatus is filled. Completely-in-the-canal (CIC) hearing aids fit down in the external auditory meatus deeply.

When orienting a client to the hearing aids, it is important to make sure she understands the components of the hearing aid as well as how to properly insert and remove the hearing aids, change the battery, and properly take care of the hearing aids. Hearing aids should be cleaned on a regular basis. Tools are provided with the hearing aids, but it is important to make sure the client knows how to use the tools. Cerumen (more commonly known as earwax) is produced in the ear canal, and even if a client has never had difficulty with cerumen before, when she begins to use hearing aids, she may notice that she has to clean cerumen from her hearing aids. Hearing aids should not get wet. That does not mean that a person cannot go out in the rain with their hearing aids in; however, the hearing aids should not be submerged in water such as in a bath, shower, or pool.

There are many adjustments that can be made to hearing aids. Many times clients do not realize or forget that it takes time to adjust to hearing sounds that have not been heard clearly for some time. Some clients also do not realize that adjustments can be made to hearing aids so that if a particular sound is causing them difficulty or they are struggling to hear certain sounds, the hearing aids may be able to be reprogrammed. Often it is important to counsel clients on realistic expectations of hearing aids. Hearing aids are different from glasses in that when you put on correctly fit glasses you see at normal vision; however, hearing aids do not cause your hearing to return to normal. Instead, they make sounds that were too soft for your hearing acuity louder. The ear may still have difficulty processing the sounds at a louder level so a person may still struggle with certain sounds or in certain situations.

As an audiologist or speech-language pathologist, you will likely encounter clients who wear hearing aids. By having a general understanding of the devices, you will be able to better assist your clients with their communication. New advances in technology are being made every day, so it is important to find a resource that provides updated information or guidance for you and your clients.

THE ACTIVITY

A. Complete the crossword puzzle in **Figure 13–1** to check your knowledge.

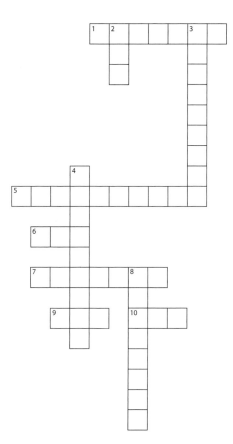

Figure 13–1 Hearing Aids Crossword Puzzle

ACROSS

1. A type of processing
5. The part of the hearing aid that picks up sound
6. Abbrev.—a hearing aid that goes behind the ear
7. The power of the hearing aid
9. Abbrev.—a hearing aid that fills the entire concha bowl
10. Abbrev.—a hearing aid that is very small and fits deeply in the canal

DOWN

2. Abbrev.—a hearing aid that covers the canal entrance
3. The part of a hearing aid that increases the sound level
4. The part of a hearing aid fitting when you teach the client to care for the hearing aid
8. The part of the hearing aid that changes the electrical signal back into an acoustic signal

B. While observing, check off the following concepts that were discussed with the client.

____ Insertion/removal   ____ Cleaning the instrument

____ Using the cleaning tools   ____ Wearing schedule

____ Parts of the instrument   ____ Battery size

____ Changing the battery   ____ Explanation of programs

____ Other—list _____

_____

_____

_____

Did the client struggle with any concepts? If so, what? Describe how that concept could have been explained differently.

_____

_____

_____

_____

C. Next, if you are observing a session where the client is returning for a hearing aid adjustment, identify the following:

Did the clinician inquire about the aid?

_____

_____

Did the clinician check the battery?

_____

_____

Did the clinician clean the hearing aid?

_____

_____

Did the clinician check the client's ear for excessive cerumen?

_____

_____

Did the clinician modify his or her own loudness or rate?

_____

_____

THE WRAP-UP

☐ *Suggestions for Reflection*

Think about the session you just observed. Did the client have realistic expectations of what the hearing aid(s) would do for him? How could you tell? Was there certain information or parts of the hearing aid with which the client seemed to have trouble? What were they and how was the information given in various ways to make sure the client understood?

_____

_____

_____

_____

What size hearing aid batteries did the hearing aid use? Did the client have any problems with changing the battery? Were there any special tools used to aid with the battery? Did she have problems with insertion/removal of the hearing aid?

_____

_____

_____

_____

◻ *Suggestions for Predictions*

Is there any information that you would give to a client regarding amplification that was not given during the session? What do you see as vital information that the client should understand before he leaves? Why that particular information?

_____

_____

_____

_____

Think about someone you know who wears hearing aids. Did he or she have a hard time adjusting to hearing aids? Why or why not? How could you assist someone with those problems?

_____

_____

_____

_____

ANSWERS

A.

ACROSS	DOWN
1. digital	**2.** ITC
5. microphone	**3.** amplifier
6. BTE	**4.** orientation
7. battery	**8.** receiver
9. ITE	
10. CIC	

CHAPTER **14**

Auditory Processing

THE FOCUS

A disorder in auditory processing is typical when there are difficulties in the way we process verbal information. The peripheral hearing is within normal limits, meaning that the person does not have difficulty hearing the level of sounds or speech (no problems with hearing sensitivity); however, when listening to speech there are problems understanding/interpreting the speech signals. For instance, a person with auditory processing problems may have a delayed response to verbal questions or he may have difficulty in the presence of background noise although he is not struggling with level of sound. Another auditory processing disorder may occur when a person can follow one- or two-step directions but cannot remember steps beyond that when directions are heard rather than read or seen.

Diagnosing auditory processing problems consists of obtaining information and test results from several different professions. It is important to be involved in a team when it comes to seeking a diagnosis for auditory processing because different professionals may see different aspects of the person's behavior depending on the setting. Some team members are parents, teachers, speech-language pathologists, audiologists, and psychologists. Typically, the audiologist will perform a battery of tests to determine the particular area or areas with which the person is struggling. The test battery the audiologist will use consists of various tasks where the client will listen to auditory information, which may include signals that may not be clear, signals that compete with one another, or signals that have varying lengths (the audiologist electronically alters the signal). The audiologist will need input from the other team members (e.g., language test scores, performance in school, difficulty with particular situations or academic areas) to incorporate with the results from the audiology and auditory processing testing in order to make sure that the diagnosis is accurate.

After the test results have been calculated, the audiologist, in collaboration with his/her colleagues, may give recommendations based on the areas of weakness the client exhibits. Some suggestions include (keep in mind this is not an exhaustive list) (1) to assist the client in the presence of background noise (preferential seating or the use of a frequency modulation system), (2) to assist with spelling or reading comprehension (some clients particularly struggle when things are not very specific so they may need to be taught the rules of spelling or how to make inferences based on a reading passage), (3) to present information in more than one modality (using visual aids along with auditory information), or (4) to teach a child to advocate for himself/herself (ask the teacher to repeat the information or assignment or even develop a visual schedule that works for him). Research is being conducted to identify new diagnostic tools and treatment recommendations for auditory processing disorders. There is no one right set of remediation suggestions for all children with auditory processing deficits; it must be individualized.

The SLP may be responsible for overseeing the implementation of the actual treatment plan recommended by the team. Therapy should consider addressing the child, the partners, and/or the environment. When the focus is on the child with auditory processing difficulties, a treatment session may look a lot like language therapy. The clinician may be working on language activities such as sequencing, language comprehension, and problem solving as the child's expressive language is often at a higher level than her receptive language. A clinician may be going over the specific rules of language such as spelling rules or sentence structure guidelines. You may also see a clinician assisting a client with organization, as this is an area of weakness for many clients with auditory processing problems, or role playing how to advocate for accommodations they require to be successful. When the focus is on the partner, you may see the clinician consulting with the teachers to help them provide clear, oral directions, use gestures, and exercise patience when a repetition of information is required. When the focus is on the environment you may see the clinician suggesting seating change; identifying especially difficult settings such as gyms, cafeterias, or open classrooms; and encouraging the use of FM systems.

Keep in mind, team collaboration is key for success when working with clients with auditory processing problems. The auditory pathway continues to mature through early adolescence, so the team members may see vast differences in a client as he ages; however, auditory processing difficulties do not go away just because a person ages. Again, communication among the team is very important to ensure the success of the client with auditory processing difficulties.

THE ACTIVITY

A. In the following scenarios, identify at least one possible recommendation in each of the focus categories of child, partner, and environment:

Scenario 1. Description of problem noted in the school: Fifth-grader whose coach found he did not follow direction in basketball practice in the gymnasium (student scored in the below average area for listening in noise).

Possible recommendation—at least one in each focus category:

1. Child

_____

_____

_____

_____

2. Partner

_____

_____

_____

_____

3. Environment

_____

_____

_____

_____

Scenario 2. Description of the problem noted in school: Third-grader leaves off parts of assignments when writing assignments in her homework folder (student scored 20 percent on auditory memory tests).

Possible recommendations—at least one in each focus category:

1. Child

_____

_____

_____

_____

2. Partner

_____

_____

_____

_____

3. Environment

_____

_____

_____

_____

Scenario 3. Description of the problem noted in school: Fourth-grader struggles with reading comprehension (student scored 40 percent on auditory memory test and 20 percent on sequencing activities).

Possible recommendations—at least one in each focus category

1. Child

_____

_____

_____

2. Partner

_____

_____

_____

_____

3. Environment

_____

_____

_____

_____

AS YOU OBSERVE...

B. From the session you observed, designated as addressing auditory processing, answer the following questions.

What was the task on which the client had the most difficulty?

_____

_____

_____

_____

What was the task on which the client had least difficulty?

_____

_____

_____

_____

Write a hypothesis concerning the role auditory processing may have played in the difficulty level of each task.

_____

_____

_____

_____

Did the clinician modify the task or talk with the client about compensatory strategies when he or she does not understand something? Explain.

_____

_____

_____

_____

What made this session stand out as addressing auditory processing?

_____

_____

_____

_____

After your observation, identify at least one thing you know about auditory processing disorders and at least one point on which you are still unclear.

_____

_____

_____

_____

THE WRAP-UP

◘ *Suggestions for Reflection*

Think about a time in your life when you did not understand the directions or missed part of the message and did not have a way to clarify. How did you feel and what steps did you take to get the missed information?

_____

_____

_____

_____

Have you ever been in a noisy environment and had difficulty hearing the specifics of conversation (even though you could tell someone was talking and you could pick out parts of what they were saying)? What was your frustration level when trying to communicate? What was your partner's level of frustration? What steps could you have taken in that situation to make it easier to communicate?

_____

_____

_____

_____

◻ *Suggestions for Prediction*

How could you work with a client who has difficulty with spelling? Are there ways that spelling tests could be given visually? If so, would that compromise the validity and reliability of the spelling test?

_____

_____

_____

_____

What information would you give to parents of a student who has been diagnosed with auditory processing, specifically with auditory memory problems? Is there a way they could move from visual cues to auditory cues to increase memory?

_____

_____

_____

_____

ANSWERS

Scenario 1. Child—Teach the child to ask for clarification when he does not hear the instructions clearly. Partner—Make sure the partner is aware of the auditory processing disorder and what it means for the child. Environment— If available, use an FM system during practices.

Scenario 2. Child—Have child take her folder to the teacher for review before leaving the class. Partner—Have the teacher write the assignments on the board. Environment—Have the child sit up close to the teacher so she has better opportunities for seeing/hearing discussion about assignments.

Scenario 3. Child—Have the child complete simple, two-step sequencing activities and then build on that foundation. Partner—Use discussion/follow-up questions to check for comprehension. Environment—Use books on tape that discuss the main ideas and concepts of the book.

The Therapy Process

CHAPTER 15

Organization of the Session

THE FOCUS

Think of the organization of a session as headings in an outline. The details or specific information under a heading will change, but the overriding topics remain similar across sessions. This is the routine of the session. Routines are important in that they help clients feel safe and allow them to anticipate the next step. They also make your job as an SLP more manageable. You know what you need to determine and plan because you know what routine you are addressing. The routine chosen is part of the clinical decision making involved in planning for an individual client. The more times you observe the same clinicians and clients working together, the easier it will be for you to identify the organization the clinician uses.

A typical routine for a pullout session might include the following:

A. Welcome and social conversation setting the stage for what will be learned
B. Review of homework and/or previous session's work
C. Identification of the day's objective and teaching the skills needed to address the objective
D. Several practice activities, perhaps varying the level of requirements, the level of structure as the session progresses, or the level of reinforcement provided
E. Review of the day's objective and outcome of the session
F. Probing for targets or levels appropriate for the next session
G. Closing

A typical routine for a whole-class session in a classroom might include the following:

A. Introductions and space/seating/materials organization

B. Identification of purpose/focus of lesson

C. Teaching the content of the lesson

D. One practice activity with multiple opportunities for practice and corrective feedback

E. Generalization of learned information to unlearned tasks or items

F. Review of learning

G. Goodbyes and return of seating/materials to original location

THE ACTIVITY

A. To identify the organization of your observed session, write the number of the appropriate details next to the appropriate heading. After you have completed your placement, check the answer key for consideration. Notice that the same task could fit under multiple headings (hint: knowing when they occur may help you with placement in the routine outline).

Match the details to the heading:

Heading

_____ A. Welcome and social conversation setting the stage for what will be learned

_____ B. Review of homework and/or previous sessions work

_____ C. Identification of the day's objective and teaching skills

_____ D. Several practice activities perhaps varying the level of requirements or the level of structure as the session progresses

_____ E. Review of day's objective and outcome of session

_____ F. Probing for next session

_____ G. Closing

Details Observed

1. playing a board game
2. naming cards
3. instruction on placement cues
4. singing a clean-up song
5. reviewing the vowel placement chart
6. trial therapy on possible things to target
7. discussing what the client did since last session
8. instruction on lip rounding for the /w/
9. conversational practice
10. examination of day's percentage scores
11. explanation of homework assignment
12. review of skill use since last session
13. probing for generalization of learning
14. talk about the weather

B. Outline the session you are observing. Make sure you include headings and specific detail under the headings. You do not need to limit yourself to the headings we have supplied. The reason for completing this activity is simple. Having a clear organization will make your therapy more consistent, your planning more efficient, and focus to teachers and families more transparent.

Outline of Observed Session's Organization

A. _____

   1. _____

   2. _____

B. _____

   1. _____

   2. _____

C. _____

   1. _____

   2. _____

D. _____

   1. _____

   2. _____

E. _____

   1. _____

   2. _____

F. _____

   1. _____

   2. _____

G. _____

   1. _____

   2. _____

H. _____

   1. _____

   2. _____

THE WRAP-UP

◻ *Suggestions for Reflection*

Consider the organization of a favorite class you have taken. Was there a routine across days? What effect did that play in your learning and liking of the class?

_____

_____

_____

_____

Did the client(s) you observed appear to know the organization of the session? Give specific examples from the session that influenced your answer. Do you think this was an asset or deficit to meeting the goals for the client(s)?

_____

_____

_____

_____

◻ *Suggestions for Prediction*

What change in organization of this session might have benefited this client? Why is organization planned?

_____

_____

_____

How might a clock with pictures of table time, snack time, story time, etc., be used to support organization of a session for a preschool child?

_____

_____

_____

What visual device might be more appropriate than the picture clock for organization of a session with an adult client?

_____

_____

_____

_____

ANSWERS

A.

A = 14

B = 5, 7

C = 2, 3, 5

D = 1, 2, 8, 9, 14

E = 10, 12

F = 6

G = 4, 11, 13

16

Online Transcription

Speech is fleeting. To capture these momentary episodes so they can be examined and analyzed, a recording, preferably with visual as well as auditory information, is extremely useful. However, there are times when a clinician relies on an online transcription, writing down verbatim the specific episode(s) of communication. This is done when recording is not possible or when a transcription is needed immediately instead of after reviewing the recording post session. An online transcription is often less accurate and less rich in contextual information than a transcribed recording of the session but can be sufficient for preliminary data collection in the following situations:

- When establishing baseline (e.g., obtaining an initial sample of the verbal messages of a child with autism as he moves around his classroom to determine functions of language used)
- When monitoring progress (e.g., collecting a biweekly sample of answers to thought-provoking questions by an adult with mild aphasia to check word finding strategies being acquired)
- When checking for generalization (e.g., taking a sample of the interaction between an adolescent with cognitive impairments and his job coach as you accompany them to the job site to determine if the pragmatic skills are being carried over).

One commonly used format for transcription has a column for the clinician's words, a column for the client's words, and a column between for contextual information deemed key in understanding the words of the clinician and client. The context includes materials (e.g., book about lions), gestures (e.g., clinician pretends to cry), and situations (e.g., person knocks on door for admittance) that enhance the interpretation of the verbal message. The contextual column is especially important to interpretation of the transcription when a speaker uses deictic terms (i.e., words where meaning changes based on the perspective of the speaker, e.g., *that, you, then,* or *there*), telegraphic utterances (i.e., sentences with content words but limited function words typical of young children's speech, e.g., "Ball table" or "Doggie jump"), or circumlocution (i.e., talking around an intended word, typically when difficulty occurs in retrieving a word from memory, e.g., "It's the one with, you know, the pointy thing") in his/her verbalization. The most valuable online transcriptions are sufficient in length to provide a representative sample, are accurate to promote the collection of reliable information, and are rich in context to allow precise interpretation of all utterances.

THE ACTIVITY

A. Find the examples of deictic terms, telegraphic speech, and circumlocution presented in the five examples provided in **Table 16–1**. A fourth column has been added to the transcription form for this purpose. For this exercise, each example is a different clinician/client pair and not a single ongoing transcription.

B. Rate your predicted skills as an orthographic transcriber based on your note-taking abilities in class by making an *X* on the following scale.

Predicted skill as transcriber:

Poor   Mighty Fine

C. Observe a therapy session and orthographically transcribe everything the clinician and client say for as long as you can. Use **Table 16–2** with clinician speech in column 1 and client speech in column 3 and context in the center column. When the speakers change, continue moving down a line even though you are in another column, to give a visual picture of the back-and-forth quality of the conversational exchange (see **Table 16–1** for a sample of the spacing). Take a short break and start again. Continue until you complete the columns below.

Rate your skills as an orthographic transcriber on amount transcribed, accuracy of transcription, and contextual richness captured.

Table 16–1 Transcription Activity Worksheet

Example Number/ Client's Age and Diagnosed Disability	Clinician	Context	Client	Identification of DT, TS, and C
1. 3 years of age; language delay	The boy is sick. He calls his mommy. He says _____.	Looking at picture book. Clinician pauses and gestures to signal turn.	Mommy sick.	
2. 15 years of age; traumatic head injury	Your cat sleeps in the kitchen?	Client began topic of pet when it was his turn to introduce a new topic of conversation to the group.	Mandy is my cat. He sleeps in the room where the stove and the place where you you keep the food cold.	
3. 6 years of age; specific language impairment	Tell me why you circled this picture.	Look at worksheet in first-grade classroom. Directions say, "Circle all the words that begin with the /b/ sound." Examine picture of a heart.	That is the picture of the thing in you that goes beat, beat, beat, beat. A beater starts with /b/.	
4. 63 years of age; Broca's aphasia	So tell me how you make a peanut butter and jelly sandwich. You don't like jelly? Not even grape jelly?	A set of four pictures depicting the steps have been put in order in front of client.	Bread. Butter bread. Jelly no. Knife cut. Eat up.	
5. 8 years of age; articulation disorder	Tell me where the x should go.	Client points to the picture and the place in the tic-tac-toe where he wants it to go.	That one goes there.	

DTs = deictic terms; TS = telegraphic speech; Cs = circumlocutions.

Table 16–2 Transcription Form

Clinician	Context	Client

Amount transcribed

```
┌──────────────────────┬──────────────────────┐
```

Little captured   Sufficient for analysis

Accuracy of transcription

```
┌──────────────────────┬──────────────────────┐
```

Many words missing or incorrect   Sample complete

Contextual richness

```
┌──────────────────────┬──────────────────────┐
```

Little identified   Important aspects included

THE WRAP-UP

◻ *Suggestions for Reflection*

Compare and contrast the skills needed in classroom note taking to the skills needed for transcription of a session.

_____

_____

_____

_____

How did transcribing affect your observation of the session? Were you more or less focused?

_____

_____

_____

_____

When might the use of deictic terms, telegraphic speech, and circumlocutions be considered acceptable, and when might it be a component of a disorder?

_____

_____

_____

_____

◻ *Suggestions for Prediction*

Consider the addition of a therapy goal-specific fourth column (e.g., correct /r/ production or inclusion of verb) to the transcription form. In the session you observed, what specific speech/language skill was the clinical focus and how could it be incorporated into the last column of the form?

_____

_____

_____

_____

What is lost if only the client's words are transcribed?

_____

_____

_____

_____

ANSWERS

A.

    1. TS (Mommy, I am sick.)

    2. C (kitchen)

    3. DT (this) and C (heart)

    4. TS (You take out the bread. Put peanut butter on it. Leave off the jelly. Use the knife to cut it. Then you eat the sandwich.)

    5. DT (that one) and DT (there).

B. Answers will vary but probably on the positive end of the rating scale.

Predicted skill as transcriber:

```
┌─────────────────────────┬──────────────────────X──────┐
```
Poor   Mighty Fine

CHAPTER 17

Ethical Behavior

Ethical behavior involves putting the welfare of the client at the heart and center of everything. Professional organizations such as the American Speech-Language-Hearing Association and the American Academy of Audiology have adopted written codes of professional conduct termed *codes of ethics* (see these organizations' Web sites to review a copy of their codes of ethics: www.asha.org/docs/html/ET2010-00309.html, www.audiology.org/resources/documentlibrary/Pages/codeofethics.aspx). Both of these organizations' codes of ethics include principles and rules to which members of their organizations aspire to conform. These codes identify guidelines that are critical to a clinician's provision of honest, caring services.

Ethical problems, issues, and dilemmas occur regularly and require clinicians to make ethical decisions. While there are sessions where an observer will hear ethical decisions being addressed (e.g., discussion of feeding options for a client with dysphagia or discussion of service delivery options), many sessions will not directly discuss critical ethical issues.

How, then, is ethical behavior evident in daily clinical sessions? Ethical behavior is evident through words and actions that convey respect and environments that are safe and secure. All the little things a clinician does daily that demonstrate respect for individuals and their rights are at the forefront of ethical behavior. Think for a minute of the list of things you would do that indicate your respect for a client. The list could include use of titles, greetings, and culturally sensitive language; selection of age-appropriate, relevant materials, techniques, and topics; projection of a courteous attitude including active listening, turn taking in conversation, and genuine attention to a communication partner's message; and consideration of time commitments in beginning and ending of the session in a timely fashion and utilizing time within the session in a planned manner. The client's safety and security are essential to the ethical clinician. This includes a safe, protected, and confidential physical and cyber environment. Consider the preparations to make a room safe and information secure. These preparations could include items such as electrical outlets covered and windows with sturdy screens, files in regulated and locked file cabinets, and encrypted/secure internet records. Lastly, ethical behavior is evident through actions that convey therapeutic purpose. When clinicians practice evidenced-based remediation, employ goal-driven techniques, and provide accurate and timely feedback, they demonstrate ethical clinical behavior.

THE ACTIVITY

A. Consider the 10 examples of disrespectful comments presented next. After each example, identify why you find it disrespectful and rewrite the clinician's words to better demonstrate respect for the client.

1. "Okay, sweetheart, that was much better this time."

_____

_____

_____

_____

2. "I don't have time to listen to your same story again."

_____

_____

_____

_____

3. "I know we started 15 minutes late, but I had important things to do."

_____

_____

_____

_____

4. "I'm sorry I don't have the handout for you but my assistant is a retard and lost it."

_____

_____

_____

_____

5. "I hadn't really thought about how we could use this game, but let's start and see where it takes us."

_____

_____

_____

_____

6. "Huh, me and Mary was figuring something out. You say something?"

_____

_____

_____

_____

7. "Let's try this. I never heard of anyone doing this and don't really think it will work, but it's worth a try."

_____

_____

_____

_____

8. "Good boy, Mr. Jones, you got that one right."

_____

_____

_____

_____

9. "I know I've asked you a million times, but what is your wife's name?"

_____

_____

_____

_____

10. "I found this great picture book with farm animals I use with another client. Mrs. Klaus, I want you to make the sound of each animal."

_____

_____

_____

_____

Consider the five examples of unsafe or unsecured environments presented in numbers 11–15. For the purposes of this activity, you are the observer at a clinical facility operating on a college campus. After each example, identify how you would address these issues right now as an ethical student observer.

11. You walk into the waiting area and almost trip on toys scattered on the floor.

_____

_____

_____

_____

12. You walk into the waiting area and find an unattended, confidential file lying open on the table.

_____

_____

_____

_____

13. You see the young client sitting quietly at the table looking through a picture book while the student clinician leaves the room for three minutes to locate forgotten material.

_____

_____

_____

_____

14. You see the young client putting small, chokable objects in his mouth while his mom and the clinician review the progress report in a corner of the room.

_____

_____

_____

_____

15. You find a draft copy of a confidential clinical report in a public copy machine in another building on campus. This is not a report from a client you have observed.

_____

_____

_____

_____

AS YOU OBSERVE…

B. List 10 statements or behaviors you observed in the session you watched that reflect clinician respect for the client or consideration of safety and security and why you selected each example (Because _____).

1. _____

_____

_____

_____

Because _____

_____

_____

_____

2. _____

_____

_____

_____

Because _____

_____

_____

_____

3. _____

_____

_____

_____

Because _____

_____

_____

_____

4. _____

_____

_____

_____

Because _____

_____

_____

_____

5. _____

_____

_____

_____

Because _____

_____

_____

_____

6. _____

_____

_____

_____

Because _____

_____

_____

_____

7. _____

_____

_____

_____

Because _____

_____

_____

_____

8. _____

_____

_____

_____

Because _____

_____

_____

_____

9. _____

_____

_____

_____

Because _____

_____

_____

_____

10. _____

_____

_____

_____

Because _____

_____

_____

_____

THE WRAP-UP

◻ *Suggestions for Reflection*

What does *ethics* mean to you? What in your background influenced your ethics?

_____

_____

_____

_____

Why do SLPs and audiologists need a code of ethics?

_____

_____

_____

_____

◻ *Suggestions for Prediction*

Will ethical dilemmas you face in remediation be easily solved by reading the code of ethics? Explain your answer.

_____

_____

_____

_____

Describe an ethical dilemma the clinician you observed might face.

_____

_____

_____

_____

Are respectful behavior and safety and security sufficient to insure that you are being ethical in your treatment? Explain your answer.

_____

_____

_____

_____

ANSWERS

A.

1. "Okay, sweetheart, that was much better this time." The term _sweetheart_ is generally not appropriate for use in a therapy session. The relationship in therapy is friendly but with some teacher–student formality present. It can also be perceived as demeaning especially if used with an adult client. Rewrite: "Okay, [inset name here], that was much better this time."

2. "I don't have time to listen to your same story again." The clinician is not listening to the client's message. If the retelling of information is getting in the way of remediation, a time could be designated when social conversation would be welcomed. Rewrite: "That reminded you of when you were on vacation. Let's finish our task and then I'd like to hear about what you did on vacation." Or the clinician could incorporate the session's goals into the topic of interest to the client. Rewrite: "I would like to hear about your vacation, but we also need to practice what we have been working on. Let's combine the two by . . ."

3. "I know we started 15 minutes late but I had important things to do." Everyone's time is important. If something has caused the clinician to be late, an apology and arrangements to make up the time are appropriate. If the clinician is late and the ses-

sion is shortened, the billing must be adjusted to charge only for the service time provided. It is unethical to bill for services not provided. Rewrite: "I apologize for being late; I had an emergency. Can we schedule a makeup time?"

4. "I'm sorry I don't have the handout for you but my assistant is a retard and lost it." The apology is appropriate. However, uses of derogatory terms are inexcusable. The clinician also needs to take responsibility for not having completed the assignment and discuss how the situation will be rectified. Rewrite: "I'm sorry I don't have the handout I promised. I will have it for you next session."

5. "I hadn't really thought about how we could use this game, but let's start and see where it takes us." Using material without a clinical focus to fill time is unacceptable. A clinician should be able to describe how any action in therapy connects to the therapeutic goals. Rewrite: "As we play this game we will be focusing on using our breathing technique. After each turn we will both rate breath support by holding up one finger if poor, two if okay, and three fingers if good."

6. "Huh, me and Mary was figuring something out. You say something?" The clinician was not courteous nor a good listener. The grammatical errors produced by the clinician were also a problem. Even if syntax is not the focus of the remediation, a clinician should always utilize grammatically correct speech. Rewrite: "I'm sorry; Mary and I were figuring out this tape and not paying attention. Would you please tell me again what you were saying?"

7. "Let's try this. I never heard of anyone doing this and don't really think it will work, but it's worth a try." This clinician is not providing evidence-based practice. The clinician needs to examine the theoretical basis and research-based evaluation of any practice used in remediation. Rewrite: "We are going to use this approach because the evidence of it working is well documented."

8. "Good boy, Mr. Jones, you got that one right." Mr. Jones is an adult and addressing him as "good boy" is inappropriate. Rewrite: "Mr. Jones, your response was correct."

9. "I know I've asked you a million times, but what is your wife's name?" The clinician needs to remember a name as important as a wife's. If the clinician cannot remember it, it should be reviewed prior to the session. If the clinician is playing a role to afford the client the opportunity to recall the name, a better

premise might be used. Rewrite: "If someone you just met asked you, 'What is your wife's name?' You would say _____."

10. "I found this great picture book with farm animals I use with another client. Mrs. Klaus, I want you to make the sound of each animal." The age appropriateness and relevance of this book and task are questionable. More pertinent material should be selected. Minimally, a context needs to be established if the clinician believes this is the appropriate level. Rewrite: "We are going to pretend you are reading this book to your granddaughter, Lucy. We will verbalize for Lucy the sound each animal makes."

11. As an observer, I would pick up the scattered material; this is about being a good community member and helping to maintain safe facilities.

12. As an observer, I would take the folder immediately to the clinical secretary or clinical supervisor on duty.

13. As an observer, I would discuss with the student clinician, after the session was concluded and the client had left, my concern about leaving any child, even one who will usually sit quietly, unattended.

14. As an observer, I would find the supervisor on duty and tell her my immediate concern.

15. As an observer, I would take the report to the clinic director and let him/her know the circumstances. Even though I know I am getting a fellow student in trouble, I would place the good of the client first. This is a breach in confidentiality and the clinical director will need to address the issue with the clinician.

CHAPTER 18

Developing Goals and Objectives

THE FOCUS

Picture a bookshelf housing all the books about communication-related skills our client strives to learn. These books represent our therapy goals and the chapters comprising each book our objectives. Goals are larger scale and inclusive while objectives are the more manageable, more narrowly defined steps taken to achieve those sought-after goals. Although it is possible to have a single volume on our hypothetical communication bookshelf, it is more common to have several volumes in need of mastery. And while the client is learning the contents of the communications shelf, he/she is also addressing the physical skill shelf, the academic knowledge shelf, etc.

Enough of this talking in riddles. Following are seven facts concerning goals and objectives:

1. Goals reflect the communication skill the client is attempting to learn. Goals often state or infer (1) the present level of functioning, (2) the level of functioning wanted, and (3) the rationale or reason for addressing the goal. An example of a goal is, *Mary will produce age-appropriate sounds during conversational speech in order to communicate effectively with family and peers.* The present level of functioning is inferred, the level wanted is stated, and the rationale is stated.

2. Goals are written following the assessment process. While standardized tests are given during assessment to help determine eligibility for services, goals are best derived from the results of interviews, observations, structured tasks, samples, and probe lists. An example of an assessment result section that facilitates goal setting follows. *Articulation testing*

revealed errors in the age-appropriate phonemes /k, g, t, and d/. Probing of each sound in error with pictures of 10 words (3 in initial position, 3 in medial position, 3 in final position, and 1 multisyllable word) revealed 10 percent accuracy for /k/, 0 percent accuracy for /g/, 30 percent accuracy for /t/, and 0 percent accuracy for /d/. A five-minute spontaneous speech sample using toys selected to elicit the error sounds resulted in accuracy consistent with probing data.

3. Goals need to be functional. Goals in the school system need to connect to academic requirements.

4. Goals can be subdivided into measurable steps needed for mastery. These steps are called objectives. Objectives are typically comprised of three parts: the doer, the deed, and the degree. Objectives build off one another to show a progression in learning. An example of a set of three objectives leading to mastery of the goal is *(1) The child will produce the age-appropriate phonemes /k, g, t, and d/ in isolation with 80 percent accuracy; (2) The child will produce the age-appropriate phonemes /k, g, t, d/ in words with 80% accuracy; and (3) The child will produce the age-appropriate phonemes /k, g, t, and d/ in sentences with 80 percent accuracy.*

5. The doer seems so obvious, yet it can lead to misunderstanding. Objectives are stated in terms of what the learner, not the clinician or teacher, will do. *Johnny will* is appropriate wording for an objective but *I will teach Johnny to* is not. The accountability movement emphasized in recent educational initiatives makes clear that what the teacher intends to teach is not necessarily learned by the pupil. We need to measure the learning.

6. The deed is the behavior to be learned. Again, this seems straightforward but can be problematic. Because we are measuring progress and ultimately mastery of the goal in terms of meeting the objectives, it is imperative that the objectives be observable, definable, and countable. The verb selected to express the deed should state an observable action. Verbs appropriate for objective use include *say, write, tell, match,* and *point to.* Verbs not appropriate for objective use include *understand, think about, consider,* and *comprehend.* All verbs are not created equal for use in behavioral objectives and the clinician should carefully select the wording.

7. The degree includes the traditional components of condition and criterion. They are combined here to reflect the interconnection between the level of accuracy expected and the level of support provided. A communication objective can be raised in difficulty by requiring production at a higher accuracy (e.g., 90 percent correct instead of 40 percent correct), or at a lesser level of support (e.g., independently instead of following a model). Some clinicians show change across objectives by increasing the accuracy required while keeping the level of support constant while others show change by maintaining accuracy level while decreasing the level of support.

THE ACTIVITY

A. Complete the seven-item question set in **Table 18–1** for the goal and objectives provided.

Sample goal 1: Tim will decrease the number of disruptive instances during P.E. class from a current level 8 a period to a level of 1 or 0 a period.

Objective 1: Given a picture outline and maximum modeling for each step, Tim will participate in P.E. class with no more than 1 outburst daily.

Objective 2: Given a picture outline and reminder of steps to follow, Tim will participate in P.E. class with no more than 1 outburst daily.

Objective 3: Given a picture outline, Tim will participate in P.E. class with no more than 1 outburst daily.

B. During your observation, state an objective the clinician appears to be addressing. Work your way backwards from the objective to the goal to the possible informal assessment activity that identified the present level of functioning. The list that follows will guide you through the steps.

1. State the objective.

The doer _____

_____

The deed _____

_____

The degree _____

_____

Put all together, the objective is _____

_____

_____

Table 18–1 Question Set for Examination of Goals and Objectives

1a	What is the present level of functioning? Is the present level inferred or stated?
1b	What is the level of functioning wanted? Is the level wanted inferred or stated?
1c	What is the rationale for the goal? Is the rationale inferred or stated?
2	What is one assessment procedure that could have led to identification of this goal (be specific)?
3	How is this goal functional or related to a specific academic goal?
4	How are the objectives related?
5	Who is the doer?
6a	What is the deed?
6b	Is the verb an appropriate observable, definable, and countable term?
7a	What is the degree?
7b	Has the clinician shown change across objectives by increasing the accuracy required while keeping the level of support constant or by maintaining the accuracy level while decreasing the level of support?

2. State the goal.

Present level of functioning _____

_____

Level of functioning wanted _____

_____

Rationale_____

_____

Connection to function or education _____

_____

Put all together, the goal is _____

_____

_____

3. State the informal assessment procedure that could have identified current functioning level. (Hint: common informal procedures include interviews, observations, structured tasks, samples, and probe lists.)

Possible procedure used _____

_____

Hypothetical data from that procedure could have been _____

_____

_____

_____

Put all together, a paragraph in the report would read _____

_____

_____

_____

THE WRAP-UP

◻ *Suggestions for Reflection*

How many goals do you think the clinician you observed addressed in the session you watched? Was this too many, not enough, or just right? Explain your answer.

_____

_____

_____

_____

List seven active verbs that might have been used to describe the objectives of the session you observed.

1. _____

2. _____

3. _____

4. _____

5. _____

6. _____

7. _____

◻ *Suggestions for Prediction*

Why are results from a normative standard test not sufficient for writing goals and objectives?

_____

_____

_____

_____

Name two communication behaviors a clinician might want to increase and two where decrease would be appropriate. Is a goal to increase a behavior better than a goal aimed at decreasing a behavior? Explain.

_____

_____

_____

_____

ANSWERS

A. The answers are shown in **Table 18–2**.

Table 18–2 Answers for Question Set for Examination of Goals and Objectives

1a	What is the present level of functioning? Is the present level inferred or stated?	8 outbursts in P.E. class a period. Stated
1b	What is the level of functioning wanted? Is the level wanted inferred or stated?	1 or fewer outbursts a P.E. period. Stated
1c	What is the rationale for the goal? Is the rationale inferred or stated?	In order to increase his learning and acceptance by peers. Inferred
2	What is one assessment procedure that could have led to identification of this goal (be specific)?	Observations and interviews with P.E. teachers were most likely used. I would have observed him in P.E. class for several days and perhaps interviewed Tim as to his perception of P.E. class.
3	How is this goal functional or related to a specific academic goal?	Social teaming is required school learning as is successful completion of P.E. class.
4	How are the objectives related?	The objective increase in difficulty by decreasing the support at each successive step. The objectives lead to the goal.

5	Who is the doer?	Tim
6a	What is the deed?	Participation in P.E. with minimal outbursts.
6b	Is the verb an appropriate observable, definable, and countable term?	Yes
7a	What is the degree?	The degree remains at 1 or less a P.E. class period, but what changes with each successive objective was the amount and type of support being provided by the clinician.
7b	Has the clinician shown change across objectives by increasing the accuracy required while keeping the level of support constant or by maintaining the accuracy level while decreasing the level of support?	Yes, by maintaining the accuracy while decreasing the support from picture outline and modeling to picture outline alone.

CHAPTER 19

Baseline

THE FOCUS

Gathering baseline data is one of the first things you will need to do with a newly diagnosed client to identify his or her current level of functioning on each objective. Baseline will give you information on how the client is doing and the level of the goals you will need to be working to achieve. Baseline data is not only taken at the beginning but at any time you want to verify that progress is being made on a particular goal.

For most articulation and language goals, you will be trying to help the client reach a higher percentage level, meaning he is getting closer to mastery of the goal. For phonologic processes and some behavior issues, you will be looking for the client to reduce the use of the process or behavior. With clients who need to increase their ability to make a certain sound or use a particular language rule, you would set your accuracy level at 80–90 percent so the targeted skill will generalize, become automatic, and require less conscious effort to produce. With phonologic processes, if the client can reduce the occurrence to less than 40 percent, it is assumed that the client is only using the process in a few instances and is in the process of mastering the rules of sounds. A targeted level for decrease in a behavior issue will vary depending on factors such as whether the behavior is injurious to self or others and time to get the behavior under control. In order to keep track of how well the client is doing, the clinician will need to obtain baseline data.

In order to get baseline data, the clinician will need to find out how many times the client makes the error out of the number of total times the particular sound was used. A good way to obtain this baseline information is to develop a list of baseline items that contain the targeted sound at the targeted level (a minimum of 10) and a few that allow you to observe generalization (3–10 at a higher level or a closely related errored sound). So if a client struggled making the /b/ sound, the clinician would need to document how many times the client made the correct /b/ sound out of the total number of possibilities. A client may have a baseline of 0 correct out of 10 opportunities, restated as 0/10 or simply 0 percent. This would indicate the client did not make the sound at any time that she had the opportunity. A clinician may find that the client is *stimulable* for the sound or that the client can make the sound in isolation when provided a model and/or cue, but when the client couples the target sound with any other sound, she cannot produce the correct target. In this case, the client may have 100% usage in isolation but 0% at the syllable level.

Goals cannot be written without knowing how well a client is doing. For this reason, baseline data should be obtained during a diagnostic session if it is determined the client will be needing services. This way, if the clinician who does the diagnostic does not continue working with the client for therapy, the new clinician will know right where to begin. Most insurance companies also require that baseline data be included with the goals when obtaining prior authorization for services. During periodic treatment sessions, the clinician will keep baseline data in order to write the subjective, objective, assessment, and plan note and compare results from treatment session to treatment session and to the accomplishment of the goal.

Remember the following when developing your baseline list:

- The purpose of a baseline list is to document change. You will refer to these items for comparison regularly, so make sure you note the list of items you used in the baseline.
- The baseline data are needed at the conclusion of the diagnostic session, especially when reimbursement is being sought.
- A baseline list typically contains between 10 and 20 items.
- At least 10 items are at the current level and the other items are to identify generalization to a higher level and to other errored but non-targeted sounds, grammatical forms, or situations.
- Baseline words are usually not worked on directly in remediation, so consider this when developing your list.
- The mode of presentation used at baseline should be maintained when baseline is readministered. Did you model the item? Did you provide a picture stimulus? Did you set it up in a cloze procedure? Did you take your information from a story retelling?
- Baseline data is not readministered every session but at intervals typically every four to six weeks so baseline is not your every session subjective, objective, assessment, and plan note data.
- The purpose of a baseline list is to document change.

THE ACTIVITY

A. Read the following scenarios and (1) determine baseline percentage data, (2) identify 5 additional baseline words you could add to reach 10 and (3) identify 5 generalization items you would add to make the total baseline list of 15 items.

Scenario 1. The goal is to correctly use /d/ in all positions of the word with 90% accuracy. This child also has errors in /g, and k, and t/.

Data: client says "bad" for *dad*, "bog" for *dog*, "ab" for *add*, "bay" for *day*, and "bot" for *dot*.

    1. _____ correct /5 = _____ percent

    2. additional baseline words (5) _____

    3. generalization items (5) = _____

Scenario 2. The goal is to reduce the occurrence of initial consonant deletion to less than 40 percent.

Data: client says "at" for *cat*, "me" for *bee*, "og" for *dog*, "ow" for *cow*, "nebra" for *zebra*, and "ear" for *bear*.

    1. _____ correct /5 = _____ percent

    2. additional baseline words (5) _____

    3. generalization items (5) _____

Scenario 3. The goal is to increase the use of spontaneous words when labeling.

Data: the client labeled *cup* and *spoon* when asked to tell what items were on the table (items on the table included cup, plate, fork, spoon, and bowl).

    1. _____ correct /5 = _____ percent

    2. additional baseline words (5) _____

    3. generalization items (5)_____

AS YOU
OBSERVE...

B. Develop a tracking form similar to the one shown in **Table 19–1** for keeping baseline (hint: you may want to keep more than one goal on a page and list your goals). Keep data on the client you are observing.

Table 19–1 Sample Tracking Form

Client: _____ Date: _____

Goal: _____

(Place Where Data Could Be Kept; i.e., + for Correct, − for Incorrect)

THE WRAP-UP

☐ *Suggestions for Reflection*

Think about the client you just observed. What was the data for today's session? Is he or she close to his or her goal?

_____

_____

_____

_____

Why is it important to keep data during every session? Is the clinician keeping data during the session? If he or she is not keeping data while the session is going, how do you think he or she is getting the data? Do you like the idea of keeping data on the spot or going back and reviewing sessions later? What are the pros/cons of each?

_____

_____

_____

_____

How does session data differ from baseline data?

_____

_____

_____

_____

Why include generalization items in your baseline data list?

_____

_____

_____

_____

Is there a way to gather baseline data during play rather than the typical list format?

_____

_____

_____

_____

◼ *Suggestions for Prediction*

What age group would be the most difficult on which to keep accurate data? Why this particular age group?

_____

_____

_____

_____

What methods may help you keep data? Will you develop your own data sheet or have you found one that you particularly like? What makes that data sheet appealing?

_____

_____

_____

_____

Explain to a parent why every other week you spend 10 minutes of your time retaking baseline data.

_____

_____

_____

_____

ANSWERS

A.

Scenario 1.

1. *80 percent.*

2. *Odd, due, dip, food, red.*

3. *Spider, radio, hot dog, bulldozer, mermaid.*

Scenario 2.

1. *40 percent.*

2. *Top, ball, fish, book, car.*

3. *I see top, I see ball, I see fish, I see book, I see car.*

Scenario 3.

1. *40 percent.*

2. *Knife, placemat, napkin, salt, pepper.*

3. *Blue cup, small plate, sharp knife, big fork.*

CHAPTER 20

Selection of Materials

THE FOCUS

When planning your sessions, you will be responsible for determining what materials you will be using with the client. This sounds like it would be the easy and fun part; however, in the beginning, it may not turn out to be as easy as it sounds. There are many factors to keep in mind when choosing materials, such as the client's age, physical ability, mental ability, goals, interests, and play skills, as well as portability, cost, and time for the session. This chapter is going to help you think through some of those issues as well as discuss staying flexible as a clinician and being able to immediately respond to your client's treatment plan.

When clinicians begin planning for clients, they typically take into consideration the goals and the age of the client. These are extremely important, but they are not the only two considerations to be made. If a client has physical limitations, he may not be able to carry out some of the activities as planned. It may take some modifications on the clinician's part to make it work for the client. For instance, if you have a client who has just been in a car accident and has two broken arms, chances are this client will not be able to perform the writing tasks that go along with some of her memory goals. Also, if you have a client who is 8 years old and working on articulation errors but also has a learning disability in reading and is learning sight words at a kindergarten level, you will not want to choose a board game that requires the client to be able to read independently to play the game. However, you may find that the client really likes board games, and so you may be able to modify the game to make it work for that client.

Some clinicians use thematic units when planning for a session. A thematic unit just means that all activities are centered around one central theme. For instance, a book that has a particular sound throughout the book could be chosen, and all activities could relate to things in the book. Some clinicians choose to have activities that are play based. In this case, the clinician may have various centers or stations with various activities that all target the same goals. The client may not realize he is doing anything other than moving from activity to activity; however, the clinician has carefully thought out the activities and makes sure that multiple opportunities for the target will be presented through each center. The clinician could also have various opportunities for the target and point out how an activity provides those opportunities. Thematic units may also be useful with a group who present a variety of goals to provide them with a common link. The theme for an adult group may be favorite foods. This would allow one member to write recipes, while another makes a list of local restaurants, and a third practices ordering from a menu. In a children's group, an endangered species unit could lead to lessons in synonyms, vocabulary targeting specific phonemes, or narrative generation.

It is always helpful if you can gather information on what the client enjoys and try to incorporate some of those activities into your session. For many clients, treatment sessions are hard work because they are asked to perform activities that are difficult for them. If you can make some of the activities align with some of their interests, you may find you have an easier time keeping that client engaged in therapy. If, during a session, you have chosen an activity and it is not working out the way you had planned or the client is getting highly frustrated and is getting to the point he wants to stop working altogether, you may need to be flexible and change your activity, take a break, or try something totally different. Consider following the client's lead on how the materials could be used. It is because of these situations that we recommend you always have several more activities than you think you need. There will be times that a client will go through an activity much faster than you anticipated or that a client dislikes a particular activity and you need a backup plan. It will be much less stressful for you and your client if you have additional activities from which to choose. If you do not need all of the prepared activities for a given session, you can save them for the next session. The important thing is to overplan rather than underplan.

Materials can be purchased from specialized education companies (e.g., articulation card packs or sequencing cards), selected from general retail stores (e.g., popular games or books), individually made by the clinician (game boards drawn in file folders or made from packs of playing cards), or gathered from the environment (magazines or items found in your purse or book bag). Cost, portability, functionality, and use across a variety of ages or for a variety of purposes are all factors to consider when selecting materials.

There are some instances when a client's behavior is a concern. It will be important to know (or learn) the difference between a client really disliking the activity and a real behavior concern. As clinicians, it can be difficult to be the person who has to institute rules and expectations. Many times, clients will push the limits to see if they can get away with something. You may have to go over expectations and rules with the client and let him know the consequences if he does not follow the rules. Supervisors are there to assist clinicians to learn to set these boundaries and also to determine if it is a true behavior concern or if there is a problem with the session plan or activities.

THE ACTIVITY

A. How could you modify the memory game for a client who seems to focus more if she is up and moving around?

_____

_____

_____

_____

B. Name five specific ways to use a grocery store newspaper advertisement with an adult language client (indicate goal area addressed and how the material would be used).

1. _____

2. _____

3. _____

4. _____

5. _____

AS YOU OBSERVE...

C. Complete the information below based on the session you are observing about four different materials used. Try to select materials that ranged in how well they appeared to work with this individual client.

1. A material used was_____ .

This material would be best for individuals from _____ to _____ years old.

This material was (check one) _____ bought from an education company; _____ bought from a retail store; _____ clinician made; or _____ found items.

This material was (check one) _____ new this session; _____ used before; _____ used every session.

This material was adopted for this specific client by _____

_____ .

This material reflected the client's interests by _____

_____ .

Name a way this material could be adapted to address a different goal:

_____

_____ .

Name a way this material could be adapted to address a different age range:

_____

_____ .

Name another way this material could be adapted to address a different physical restriction:

_____

_____ .

The client directed the way this material was used in part by

_____

_____ .

This material was used for about _____ minutes, and that was (select one) _____ too long; _____ too short; or _____ just about the right amount of time.

2. A material used was_____ .

This material would be best for individuals from _____ to _____ years old.

This material was (check one) ____ bought from an education company; ____ bought from a retail store; ____ clinician made; or ____ found items.

This material was (check one) ____ new this session; ____ used before; ____ used every session.

This material was adopted for this specific client by _____

_____ .

This material reflected the client's interests by _____

_____ .

Name a way this material could be adapted to address a different goal:

_____

_____ .

Name a way this material could be adapted to address a different age range:

_____

_____ .

Name another way this material could be adapted to address a different physical restriction:

_____

_____ .

The client directed the way this material was used in part by

_____

_____ .

This material was used for about ____ minutes, and that was (select one) ____ too long; ____ too short; or ____ just about the right amount of time.

3. A material used was_____.

This material would be best for individuals from ____ to ____ years old.

This material was (check one) ____ bought from an education company; ____ bought from a retail store; ____ clinician made; or ____ found items.

This material was (check one) ____ new this session; ____ used before; ____ used every session.

This material was adopted for this specific client by _____

_____.

This material reflected the client's interests by _____

_____.

Name a way this material could be adapted to address a different goal:

_____

_____.

Name a way this material could be adapted to address a different age range:

_____

_____.

Name another way this material could be adapted to address a different physical restriction:

_____

_____.

The client directed the way this material was used in part by

_____

_____.

This material was used for about ____ minutes, and that was (select one) ____ too long; ____ too short; or ____ just about the right amount of time.

4. A material used was_____ .

This material would be best for individuals from ____ to ____ years old.

This material was (check one) ____ bought from an education company; ____ bought from a retail store; ____ clinician made; or ____ found items.

This material was (check one) ____ new this session; ____ used before; ____ used every session.

This material was adopted for this specific client by _____

_____ .

This material reflected the client's interests by _____

_____ .

Name a way this material could be adapted to address a different goal:

_____

_____ .

Name a way this material could be adapted to address a different age range:

_____

_____ .

Name another way this material could be adapted to address a different physical restriction:

_____

_____ .

The client directed the way this material was used in part by

_____

_____ .

This material was used for about ____ minutes, and that was (select one) ____ too long; ____ too short; or ____ just about the right amount of time.

THE WRAP-UP

◻ *Suggestions for Reflection*

Think about the session you just observed. How many materials were used in the session? Was this number sufficient? Did the clinician run out of time or materials?

_____

_____

_____

_____

Develop a material and an activity for the session you just observed.

_____

_____

_____

_____

◻ *Suggestions for Prediction*

Consider various materials you have observed in use or those you have created. Is there a better time in a session to complete certain activities (such as table work versus games)? Give your reasoning.

_____

_____

_____

_____

How will you determine if a material seems to be working? What will you do if the material is not working the way you had planned?

_____

_____

_____

_____

What would be the value in following the child's lead in material usage? When would this not be a good idea?

_____

_____

_____

_____

ANSWERS

A. The memory game could be modified for an active child by (1) taping the items to be remembered around the room; (2) doing a gesture for each item to be remembered; or (3) standing in a different corner of the room for each item to be remembered.

B. A grocery store newspaper advertisement could be used to address (1) reading by having the client read product names, (2) planning by selecting three items and having the client plan her route through the store to get the items, (3) writing by listing items to purchase with the ad serving as visual model or words, (4) a discussion by explaining personal likes and dislikes of certain items or brands, and (5) sorting by separating the coupons based on food categories.

CHAPTER 21

Session Characteristics: Speaker Dominance, Naturalness, and Attention

THE FOCUS

Dichotomies are frequently used to help us think about the parameters of an experience. Rating on a scale where endpoints are identified as dichotomies (such as good vs. bad, temporary vs. permanent, or treatment vs. assessment) can be used to help focus our attention as observers on specific characteristics. Dichotomies reflecting the concepts of speaker dominance, naturalness, and attention are characteristics of a session within the clinician's control. These characteristics are not static but rather change throughout the session.

Speaker dominance: Who is taking more and longer verbal turns? There is not a right or wrong to speaker dominance. It clearly is related to what is being taught and the method used to teach. A clinician reading an auditory bombardment list of words to focus attention on a sound target would be rated as "therapist monologue on the speaker dominance scale," while an adult client describing the steps used to make a sandwich would be scored as "client monologue."

```
┌──────────────────┬────────────────────────────┐
```

Therapist monologue   Client monologue

Naturalness: Is the activity being done, something the client typically does or is it something artificial designed to make a point or provide optimum opportunities for practice? Naturalness is related to factors such as participants (e.g., a mom is more natural than a clinician as a communication partner), setting (e.g., home is more natural than a segregated room), and materials (e.g., books are more natural than flash cards). Again, there is not a right or wrong to the degree of naturalness in a session. Some sessions are organized to begin on the artificial end of the continuum and move toward the typical end by session's conclusion.

Contrived/artificial   Natural/typical

Attention: Is the focus of the clinician or client on target or off target for the goal? The same behavior may be judged in either end of the continuum depending on the context/connection to the therapy goal. A child hiding under the table would be rated "unfocused" if he was being asked to join in carpet time but "focused" if taking part in a hiding game.

Unfocused   Focused

THE ACTIVITY

A. Rate the 10 descriptions below on the 3 scales. Compare your scoring with the answers provided. Where you have disagreement with the answer, consider what additional information you needed to have your answer match ours.

1. Description: An adult client, while using good breath support, explains which coupons from the paper he would use when grocery shopping.

Therapist monologue   Client monologue

Artificial   Natural

Unfocused   Focused

2. Description: An adolescent states the four speech fluency rules.

Therapist monologue   Client monologue

```
┌─────────────────│─────────────────┐
```
Artificial   Natural

```
┌─────────────────│─────────────────┐
```
Unfocused   Focused

3. Description: The clinician and a child converse while building with play dough but the child is into the play to the exclusion of speech.

```
┌─────────────────│─────────────────┐
```
Therapist monologue   Client monologue

```
┌─────────────────│─────────────────┐
```
Artificial   Natural

```
┌─────────────────│─────────────────┐
```
Unfocused   Focused

4. Description: The clinician models a word and the child repeats it.

```
┌─────────────────│─────────────────┐
```
Therapist monologue   Client monologue

```
┌─────────────────│─────────────────┐
```
Artificial   Natural

```
┌─────────────────│─────────────────┐
```
Unfocused   Focused

5. Description: The clinician and child sing the cleanup song as they put away materials.

```
┌─────────────────│─────────────────┐
```
Therapist monologue   Client monologue

Artificial | Natural

Unfocused | Focused

6. Description: The client describes her home assignment to her mom following a prompt by the clinician.

Therapist monologue | Client monologue

Artificial | Natural

Unfocused | Focused

7. Description: A client with English as a second language reads a list of words for speed and accuracy but has many errors.

Therapist monologue | Client monologue

Artificial | Natural

Unfocused | Focused

8. Description: The clinician reads an auditory bombardment list with slight amplification to a client who is coloring a picture as she listens.

Therapist monologue | Client monologue

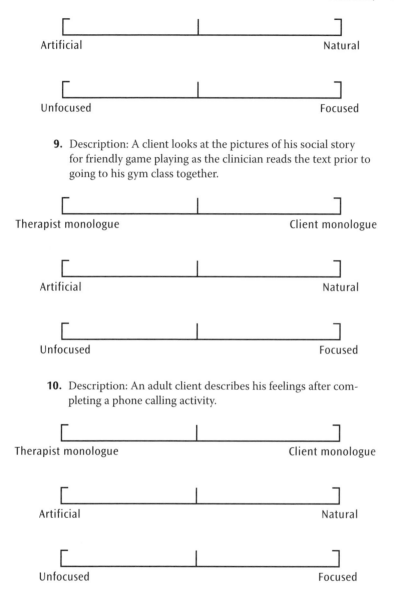

Artificial ⌐_____|_____⌐ Natural

Unfocused ⌐_____|_____⌐ Focused

9. Description: A client looks at the pictures of his social story for friendly game playing as the clinician reads the text prior to going to his gym class together.

Therapist monologue ⌐_____|_____⌐ Client monologue

Artificial ⌐_____|_____⌐ Natural

Unfocused ⌐_____|_____⌐ Focused

10. Description: An adult client describes his feelings after completing a phone calling activity.

Therapist monologue ⌐_____|_____⌐ Client monologue

Artificial ⌐_____|_____⌐ Natural

Unfocused ⌐_____|_____⌐ Focused

AS YOU OBSERVE...

B. Bring a stopwatch or clock to the session you are observing. After every five minutes of the session you are watching, note in a one-sentence description what is happening at that moment in the session and rate what is happening on the three scales of speaker dominance, naturalness, and attention.

Time 0:05 Description: _____

Therapist monologue   Client monologue

Artificial   Natural

Unfocused   Focused

Time 0:10 Description: _____

Therapist monologue   Client monologue

Artificial   Natural

Unfocused   Focused

Time 0:15 Description: _____

Therapist monologue   Client monologue

Artificial   Natural

Unfocused   Focused

Time 0:20 Description: _____

```
┌──────────────────┬──────────────────┐
```
Therapist monologue   Client monologue

```
┌──────────────────┬──────────────────┐
```
Artificial   Natural

```
┌──────────────────┬──────────────────┐
```
Unfocused   Focused

Time 0:25 Description: _____

```
┌──────────────────┬──────────────────┐
```
Therapist monologue   Client monologue

```
┌──────────────────┬──────────────────┐
```
Artificial   Natural

```
┌──────────────────┬──────────────────┐
```
Unfocused   Focused

Time 0:30 Description: _____

```
┌──────────────────┬──────────────────┐
```
Therapist monologue   Client monologue

```
┌──────────────────┬──────────────────┐
```
Artificial   Natural

```
┌──────────────────┬──────────────────┐
```
Unfocused   Focused

Time 0:35 Description: _____

Therapist monologue	Client monologue

Artificial	Natural

Unfocused	Focused

Time 0:40 Description: _____

Therapist monologue	Client monologue

Artificial	Natural

Unfocused	Focused

Time 0:45 Description: _____

Therapist monologue	Client monologue

Artificial	Natural

Unfocused	Focused

Time 0:50 Description: _____

Therapist monologue   Client monologue

Artificial   Natural

Unfocused   Focused

Time 0:55 Description: _____

Therapist monologue   Client monologue

Artificial   Natural

Unfocused   Focused

Time 0:60 Description: _____

Therapist monologue   Client monologue

Artificial   Natural

Unfocused   Focused

THE WRAP-UP

◻ Suggestions for Reflection

Summarize what you observed on the three scales of speaker dominance, naturalness, and attention.

_____

_____

_____

_____

How did the three scales change as the session progressed?

_____

_____

_____

_____

Was there a relationship among the three scales or were they independent of each other?

_____

_____

_____

_____

◻ Suggestions for Prediction

Identify another scale, including the dichotomized endpoints, that is important in capturing the structure of the session you observed. Justify the importance of your new scale.

Scale name: _____

┌_____|_____┐

Endpoints: _____   _____

In your opinion, what is the ideal place to score on the speaker dominance continuum. Why?

_____

_____

_____

_____

Identify one new activity the clinician could plan that would be at the "natural" end of the naturalness continuum.

_____

_____

_____

_____

Name something that helps a client focus on the therapy goal.

_____

_____

_____

_____

ANSWERS

A.

  1. Description: An adult client using good breath support explains which coupons from the paper he would use when grocery shopping.

```
Therapist monologue                    X        Client monologue
```

```
Artificial              X                        Natural
```

```
Unfocused                                     X  Focused
```

2. Description: An adolescent states the four speech fluency rules.

```
[_____|_____X]
Therapist monologue                    Client monologue
```

```
[X_____|_____]
Artificial                             Natural
```

```
[_____|_____X]
Unfocused                              Focused
```

3. Description: The clinician and a child converse while building with play dough, but the child is into the play to the exclusion of speech.

```
[ X_____|_____]
Therapist monologue                    Client monologue
```

```
[_____|_____X__]
Artificial                             Natural
```

```
[X_____|_____]
Unfocused                              Focused
```

4. Description: The clinician models a word and the child repeats it.

```
[_____X____|_____]
Therapist monologue                    Client monologue
```

```
[X_____|_____]
Artificial                             Natural
```

```
[_____|_____X__]
Unfocused                              Focused
```

5. Description: The clinician and child sing the cleanup song as they put away materials.

```
┌──────────────────────┬ X ──────────────────┐
```
Therapist monologue   Client monologue

```
┌──────────────────────┬── X ───────────────┐
```
Artificial   Natural

```
┌──────────────────────┬────────── X ──────┐
```
Unfocused   Focused

6. Description: The client describes her home assignment to her mom following a prompt by the clinician.

```
┌────────── X ─────┬────────────────────┐
```
Therapist monologue   Client monologue

```
┌──────────────────────┬── X ───────────────┐
```
Artificial   Natural

```
┌──────────────────────┬────────── X ──────┐
```
Unfocused   Focused

7. Description: A client with English as a second language reads a list of words for speed and accuracy but has many errors.

```
┌──────────────────────┬────────── X ──────┐
```
Therapist monologue   Client monologue

```
┌ X ───────────────────┬──────────────────┐
```
Artificial   Natural

```
┌──────────────────────┬────────── X ──────┐
```
Unfocused   Focused

8. Description: The clinician reads an auditory bombardment list with slight amplification to a client who is coloring a picture as she listens.

```
┌X                    |                        ┐
```
Therapist monologue   Client monologue

```
┌X                    |                        ┐
```
Artificial   Natural

```
┌                     |            X          ┐
```
Unfocused   Focused

9. Description: A client looks at the pictures of his social story for friendly game playing as the clinician reads the text prior to going to his gym class together.

```
┌X                    |                        ┐
```
Therapist monologue   Client monologue

```
┌  X                  |                        ┐
```
Artificial   Natural

```
┌                     |            X          ┐
```
Unfocused   Focused

10. Description: An adult client describes his feelings after completing a phone calling activity.

```
┌                     |      X                ┐
```
Therapist monologue   Client monologue

```
┌              X      |                        ┐
```
Artificial   Natural

```
┌                     |            X          ┐
```
Unfocused   Focused

CHAPTER **22**

Reinforcement

In order to keep clients motivated, it is often helpful to use reinforcement. Reinforcement can be given in a positive or negative way. Positive reinforcement is providing feedback (verbally or using objects) in a way that rewards the client for her performance. When using positive reinforcement, the clinician should determine the level at which the client needs reinforcing. For example, a very young client may need reinforcement after every correct attempt, whereas an older child or adult client may need reinforcement only after every activity is completed or possibly even at the end of the session. Positive reinforcement should only be given when there is an attempt at which the client correctly performs the activity. In a situation where the clinician would like the client to request an object by making a verbal attempt, it would not be correct to give the client the object if he pointed to the object without any verbalization.

It is also common for clinicians to want to encourage a client, thus providing positive reinforcement even when a correct attempt has not been made. Many times clinicians will nod their head or say, "Good job," even when the client has not made a correct attempt at the targeted goal. It is very important to make sure as a clinician you are providing positive reinforcement only when a correct attempt has been made. Do not be afraid to let the client know that the attempt she made was not on target. In a situation in which a client needs feedback after every attempt, the clinician should make sure he is giving specific feedback (as in the pointing example used earlier, the clinician could say, "That was a good point, but if you want to play with the ball, I need to hear you say, 'ball.'"). Being specific about feedback is important so the client is not getting mixed messages on what she is doing correctly or incorrectly.

Negative reinforcement is adjusting a behavior to avoid a negative consequence. This is different from punishment because when a punishment occurs it is a consequence to a behavior. With negative reinforcement, the client would be avoiding something negative by altering his behavior. For instance, if a clinician was trying to get a client to request objects and the clinician was using food as part of the lesson, the clinician might eat in front of the client until the client requests food. When the client learns that she can get food and avoid having to watch someone eat something she desires just by requesting the object, she can avoid the negative consequence. Using negative reinforcement is not the most common reinforcement method typically used in treatment, but it can be an effective tool.

New clinicians often find reinforcement is more difficult than they anticipated. Giving specific feedback and determining the level of reinforcement needed is not always an easy task. Generally, new clinicians want to make their clients feel good and keep trying tasks that may be hard for them; therefore they may give head nods or other forms of affirmation when it is not appropriate. By recording sessions and reviewing them later, clinicians will have the opportunity of doing some self-reflection and critique to see if they are giving mixed signals to their client.

Following are several common forms of positive reinforcement and a cautionary note for utilization of each in intervention.

1. *Verbal reinforcement.* Verbal reinforcement is a familiar form of reinforcement. Clinicians are heard to utter such accolades as *great, fantastic, good, wonderful,* and *nice talking.* One caution here concerns overuse. Even something that is pleasant and enjoyable the first, second, or third time may lose its reinforcement value when overused. Be careful not to become the "good clinician" who says the word after each production the client makes. The "good" becomes a conversation filler like "um" or "oh" rather than a means to reward or provide valuable feedback. With verbal reinforcement, the inflection with which it is delivered is also crucial, and the right inflection helps keep a word meant to reinforce from becoming an empty filler.

2. *Natural reinforcement.* In recent years, SLPs have become aware that the response to the communication itself is a terrific reinforcement. What could be better than getting that drink of juice you requested? Clinicians extend the occurrence of natural reinforcements by manipulating the environment to increase the likelihood of opportunities. They place desired items in sight but out of reach, provide portions of requested items instead of the whole thing, and act confused to increase communication opportunities that can then be rewarded naturally. A caution here is not trusting the natural reinforcement and adding verbal reinforcements on top, thus making the interaction more instructional feeling and less natural in tone.

3. *Food reinforcement.* Food can be a powerful reinforcement, and it is not uncommon to see cereal, crackers, and candy used in treatment. It is generally not the reinforcement of first choice for most SLPs for several reasons. Since we are often modifying a verbal production in speech-language therapy, food in the mouth can slow down or distort the response. Food allergies and sugar reactions are also a concern, and parental permission should always be obtained before food is given to children. Increases in obesity and diabetes in the society also make a responsible clinician consider other reinforcement options.

4. *Tangible reinforcement.* Clinicians will often reward a client by providing pieces of a puzzle, turns in a game, or stamps/stickers following a response or set of responses during a drill practice task. Care should be taken so the reinforcement does not take too much time away from the practice. As a rule of thumb, the less complicated and time consuming the tangible reinforcement, the better.

5. *Nonverbal reinforcement.* A smile, a high five, and a pat on the back can all function as nonverbal reinforcement. However, clinicians must be aware that some individuals with speech, language, or hearing disorders have difficulty perceiving or interpreting facial expressions and thus might not read that smile as it was intended. Awareness of age appropriateness of nonverbal actions such as clapping, hugging, and high fiving is important. These gestures are not equally appropriate through the life span.

THE ACTIVITY

A. Read the following scenarios and determine if reinforcement is used appropriately.

1. *The target is:* The client will correctly produce /m/ in the initial position of words. The client and clinician are going to make chocolate milk. The clinician says, "We are going to make chocolate milk. Here is your chocolate powder, your cup, and your spoon. What else do you need?" The client says, "Mil." The clinician hands the child the milk and says, "Good job. Yes, we need the milk to make the chocolate milk."

_____

_____

_____

_____

2. *The target is*: The client will put the events of a familiar routine in the appropriate sequence. The clinician gives the client three picture cards showing a series of flower-planting events. The client puts the picture cards in the following sequence: digging a hole, watering, and planting the seeds. The clinician says, "Yes, that is great. You got that right except that these last two should be switched."

_____

_____

_____

_____

3. *The target is*: The client will determine when sounds are alike or different. The clinician says, "/b/, /p/." The client says, "Different." The clinician nods his head yes and says, "/t/, /d/." The client says, "Different." The clinician nods his head and says, "/g/, /k/." The client says, "Same." The clinician nods his head and says, "Close."

_____

_____

_____

_____

B. Circle T for true and F for false before the 10 statements that follow. Then give a reason for the answers you identified as false. Check your answers and reasoning with ours.

1. T / F   Food should always be the reinforcement of choice because it works so well.

Reason: _____

_____

2. T / F   There are no appropriate nonverbal reinforcements for use with adults.

Reason: _____

_____

3. T / F   Any reinforcement can lose its potency when overused.

Reason: _____

_____

4. T / F   A piece of candy given before the production would not be considered a reinforcement for that production.

Reason: _____

_____

5. T / F   You can never be too rich or say "Good" too often.

Reason: _____

_____

6. T / F   Stringing a bead would be a good choice of a reinforcement of speech production for a child with communication and fine motor disorders.

Reason: _____

_____

7. T / F   A thumbs-up gesture would be classified as a nonverbal reinforcement type.

Reason: _____

_____

8. T / F   Softly rubbing the child's arm after a correct production would be a great reinforcement for a child who is excessively tactile defensive because it would allow the child and clinician to work on two goals at once—increasing communication and decreasing tactile defensiveness.

Reason: _____

_____

9. T / F   A smile is always a positive reinforcer.

Reason: _____

_____

10. T / F   The clinician needs to carefully consider the reinforcement he or she utilizes.

Reason: _____

_____

C. Complete **Table 22–1** based on five 5-minute time period observations. These should be spread out throughout the session observed. For each time period, record a brief description of the activity, estimated frequency of the each type of reinforcement used (V = verbal, N = natural, F = food, T = tangible, and NV = nonverbal) and a comment on the pattern of reinforcement you observed. Comments could include perceived effectiveness of the reinforcement, awareness of our cautions, or/and a rationale for use of this type of reinforcement to accomplish the goal.

THE WRAP-UP

◻ *Suggestions for Reflection*

After observing the client, determine how often the client seems to need reinforcement in order to stay motivated. Choose one activity and keep track using a +/– system to determine when reinforcement was used appropriately.

_____

_____

_____

_____

Think about a situation in which you have been given mixed messages. What made that particular reinforcement helpful? What could have been done differently to give you a better idea of your true performance?

_____

_____

_____

_____

Table 22–1 Reinforcement Observation Form

Brief Description of Activity	Estimated Frequency of the Five Types of Reinforcement					Comment on Pattern of Reinforcement
	V	N	F	T	NV	
First 5-minute time period						
Second 5-minute time period	V	N	F	T	NV	
Third 5-minute time period	V	N	F	T	NV	
Fourth 5-minute time period	V	N	F	T	NV	
Fifth 5-minute time period	V	N	F	T	NV	

Think about the session you just observed. Come up with an activity that would target the same goals. Determine if you will use positive or negative reinforcement and describe how you would use that reinforcement during your activity.

_____

_____

_____

_____

What are reinforcements for you? Name a verbal, natural, food, tangible, and nonverbal reinforcement you have used to self-reinforce (e.g., if I read one more chapter I can ...).

Why as a clinician is it important to be aware of your own reinforcement tendencies?

_____

_____

_____

_____

◻ Suggestions for Prediction

In what situations may it be more difficult for a clinician to not give reinforcement?

_____

_____

_____

_____

Think about your personality and how you respond when dealing with children and adults. How will you do as far as giving appropriate reinforcement?

_____

_____

_____

ANSWERS

A.

    1. Yes.

    2. The clinician should either say, "Great try" or leave the "Yes" off.

    3. The clinician should not nod his head after the third attempt.

B.

    1. False. Reason: Food may be an appropriate choice, but not always. Food may interfere with clear production and cautions about allergies and obesity should be considered.

    2. False. Reason: Reinforcement is always individualized. Pats on the shoulder or a touch on the hand can be appropriate for adults.

    3. True.

    4. False. Reason: Reinforcement occurs after the production, not before.

    5. False. Reason: *Good* can be said so often that it becomes a filler and may even become an annoyance.

    6. False. Reason: For this child, stringing a bead is probably a slow, difficult task and probably not the best choice of an uncomplicated and minimally time-consuming reinforcement.

    7. True.

    8. False. Reason: It is doubtful that softly rubbing this child's arm would be reinforcing after a correct production. This is equivalent to saying, "If you do something right, we will then do something you really hate."

    9. False. Reason: No, it is only a reinforcer if it increases the occurrence of the preceding behavior.

    10. True.

CHAPTER 23

Family

As clinicians and future speech-language pathologists, you will need to develop some strategies for working with family members of your clients. It is important to remember that although you understand what you are doing and the reason behind it, to others it may not seem so clear. Most family members learn as they accompany their loved ones to diagnostic or treatment sessions. They may not have any prior knowledge of speech and/ or language disorders or how they can assist the client with these disorders.

When talking with family members, you will need to remember that terms we use (especially some of our acronyms) are not always familiar to everyone. As you are thinking about ways to discuss issues with family members, it may be helpful if you think back to a time when you were not familiar with all the terms and determine what was helpful when someone was explaining them to you. For instance, rather than saying, "Your father is exhibiting aphasia due to his TBI," you may want to say something like, "Your father is having some problems with saying the word he intends to say. This is not uncommon after a traumatic brain injury such as a car accident." It is not that you want to talk down to family members or act in a way that suggests they do not understand what you are talking about, but that you want to make sure that you are using language that is common to many listeners.

You may also need to discuss the activities you worked on during the session. With adult clients, it may look as if you are doing nothing more than talking about everyday events, when in actuality you may be working on memory issues. With children it may seem as if you and the child are playing with no true focus, so it is very important to explain to the parents that you have set up activities that incorporate the targets for the child's goals. It is important that loved ones understand the activities during treatment sessions in order for them to help the client implement the strategies every day. This will assist with carryover of information as well as provide an outside source of information on how the client is doing when not in therapy and what particular issues she faces on an everyday basis. While the client is your primary focus, it is important to remember that making a connection to family members is another role you take on as a therapist.

As a clinician, you will need to know when written feedback is needed and when verbal feedback is needed. Written feedback can describe specific details of how the client is doing and if there is a particular activity you would like her to work on before the next session, as well as provide information that she and a family member can discuss together. Written feedback may also give you a chance to summarize the treatment session with the client as you are writing the note and discuss specific strategies. This is also helpful if you have appointments directly following a session; it allows you to have communication with the family member without having to take additional time before your next session. Verbal feedback certainly has a place and helps you to establish rapport with the client and family members. The same information can be given verbally; however, the client and family member will not have written information that they can refer back to before your next session.

There may be situations that are hard to discuss with family members. Occasionally, you may see a client who has more extenuating circumstances which have not been officially identified, and you may be the one to give the family additional information or make the referrals to the appropriate agencies. There will be times when this information may be very difficult for family members to hear, and you will want to develop some strategies for bringing up subjects. For instance, you may see that a client is having more difficulty with memory and may be concerned that the client is exhibiting traits more characteristic of Alzheimer's disease than dementia. This information may be very difficult for the family so you may have to start by pointing out specific things that are occurring that do not fit the dementia diagnosis. Another example could be if you are working with a child who is exhibiting signs of pervasive developmental disorder, otherwise known as being on the autism spectrum. The family may not be ready to hear that information, and it may be a case that you have to take slowly by pointing out some specific characteristics that are concerning or are more than just a language delay.

As clinicians, you are not just working with a client for a particular set time. You also have to develop relationships with family members and friends who may accompany the clients to sessions. If you are working in a setting where you do not get the opportunity to interact with the client's family members and friends, you will still need to network with them (or others such as teachers) to make sure the client is learning to use the strategies you work on outside the therapy room.

THE ACTIVITY

A. Rewrite the following statements to make them more clear to the average listener.

   1. Your child has an expressive language delay. In order to assist her, we are going to implement some strategies through structured play to increase her use of "wh" questions.

_____

_____

_____

_____

   2. Mr. Sutton is exhibiting short-term memory deficits likely due to his most recent stroke. I have also noticed that he seems to be having some dysphagia. Has that been addressed by his physician?

_____

_____

_____

_____

   3. Sally is exhibiting signs of apraxia. I am recommending the use of an AAC device to assist with her communication until we develop some strategies to help with her speech.

_____

_____

_____

_____

B. Develop a form to provide written documentation to the family. Do not forget important information such as the date, progress, and activities to work on before the next session.

AS YOU
OBSERVE... **C.** As you watch the session, identify two places where a description or explanation would be helpful to the family. Write those descriptions or explanations in family-friendly language.

1. _____

_____

_____

_____

2. _____

_____

_____

_____

AS YOU OBSERVE... **D.** Complete the written documentation form you have devised in step B based on the session you are observing.

THE WRAP-UP

□ *Suggestions for Reflection*

Think of the session you just observed. Did the clinician speak with the family member before or after the session? What information was relayed to the family member? What did you see as an observer that lacked clarity? List something specific that occurred during the session that you feel would need to be explained to the family member. How would you explain it?

_____

_____

_____

_____

Do you like giving written or verbal information or a combination? Why is that your preference?

_____

_____

_____

_____

◻ *Suggestions for Prediction*

What situation do you perceive as being a hard one to talk about with family members?

_____

_____

_____

_____

How do you broach subjects with family members that they do not want to discuss?

_____

_____

_____

_____

Write a script of how you would talk with a mother about working with a 9-year-old child with a lisp when you note his mom also has this articulation error.

_____

_____

_____

_____

ANSWERS

A.

   1. Test results show that your child understands more things than she says. For instance, she could point to the correct picture when asked, "Where is the horse?" but did not ask many questions. In order to help with this, I am going to set up some activities that will give her opportunities to ask questions. The activities will look like we are just playing with some farm animals, but they will be centered around her having opportunities to ask questions.

   2. Mr. Sutton seems to be having some trouble with his short-term memory. I am seeing this when we talk about something and then I ask him some questions about what we have just discussed and he cannot remember all the parts. I know he recently had a stroke and it is not uncommon to have these problems following a stroke. I am noticing that he also seems to be having a hard time swallowing his food and drink. Did they test his swallow before he left the hospital?

   3. Sally seems to be having problems with consistently saying certain speech sounds. This is sometimes called "apraxia" and means that although Sally knows what sounds she wants to say, there is a breakdown in what her brain is telling her to say and what sounds her tongue, lips, and mouth actually produce. This can be very frustrating and while we will be working on strategies to help with this, in the meantime I would like to look into some assistive technology devices that she can use. There are items like pictures she can point to or even small electronic devices that she can use that will say the word for her.

B. Sample form

Name:	Date:

What we are working on:

Data:

What should be done before our next session:

CHAPTER **24**

Supervision

THE FOCUS

Supervision is a specialized form of teaching. A supervisor is responsible for the learning of both the client and the supervisee, establishing and maintaining positive interpersonal relationships, facilitating supervisee education through a variety of teaching techniques including modeling, inquiry, and discussion, and providing the feedback to promote supervisee growth. Supervisory feedback initially comes from an outsider, the supervisor, providing advice on strengths, limitations, and suggestions for next steps. Ultimately it becomes the insider, the clinician, who independently self-critiques or self-supervises. Outside supervisors vary in the approach they take to facilitate the growth of the supervisee. Some provide written observations and suggestions, some provide their feedback orally during conferences, and some use a combination of the two. Some supervisory feedback is descriptive (e.g., *okay* was overused) while other feedback provides quantified data (e.g., *okay* was said 20 times in a five-minute period). Some feedback is in the form of a statement (e.g., "Good use of age-appropriate books"), while other feedback is in the form of a question (e.g., "How can the tasks presented in drill be moved to a more functional activity to encourage generalization?"). Feedback helps identify the clinician's strengths and limitations. While supervisees have a tendency to focus on the limitations provided and to ignore the strengths noted, noting both strengths to make even stronger and weaknesses to improve upon are critical to growth. The real value of feedback is its role in a plan of how to proceed in the future. Realizing that the supervisor's job and ultimately the supervisee's job are to critique performance and act on that critique may allow the student clinician to keep the comments in perspective.

In most training programs, a student clinician will have an opportunity to gain from the experience of working with several supervisors during the training experience. This variety will afford the clinician the opportunity to experience differing styles, perspectives, and approaches. This is a wonderful opportunity to develop a one-on-one relationship with a certified clinician. By the conclusion of training, most supervisees will have a favorite supervisor, one with whom they connected especially well. While a favorite supervisor is a good thing, it is important to learn from experiences with all of your supervisors. A respectful attitude, strong work ethic with timely completion of tasks, and willingness to communicate by actively listening and speaking with your supervisor go a long way in developing a satisfactory working relationship.

THE ACTIVITY

A. Place the letter of the feedback example (a to h) in the correct numbered boxes (1 to 8) in **Table 24–1**. Supervisors often have a focus category they are emphasizing while they evaluate. For the purpose of this exercise, the clinician's verbal and nonverbal behaviors will be evaluated. After you place each item in the appropriate box, complete the last column with your plan of how this feedback could be used to influence clinician performance during the next session. Compare your answers with the ones we provided in **Table 24–3**.

B. As you watch a session, write evaluative feedback of the verbal and nonverbal behaviors of the clinician you are observing. Put at least one example in each of the boxes of **Table 24–2**.

THE WRAP-UP

☐ *Suggestions for Reflection*

Describe a meaningful situation where you were provided with feedback on your strengths and a second one when you were provided with feedback on limitations. Which was more helpful?

_____

_____

_____

_____

Table 24–1 Supervision Activity Worksheet

a. "Wait time after asking a question did not appear sufficient for this bicultural child."
b. "The comparison of /p/ and /b/ as being made in different places of articulation was inaccurate."
c. "How could the room be better arranged so family members observing can see the child?"
d. "Was your extremely rapid rate of speech facilitative to decreasing the rate of the client's speech?"
e. "Directions for homework were clearly written on the homework sheet."
f. "Were you as comfortable as you looked when you gave the mom the results of the assessment?"
g. "Your speech was at an appropriate level—just one step higher than the client's target."
h. "Where else could your pausing be used to increase the number of accurate responses like it was in the book activity?"

Feedback Form: Strength/Limitation Statement/Question	Verbal Behavior	Nonverbal Behavior	Your Plan for Using This Information to Improve	
			Verbal	Nonverbal
Strength statement	1.	2.		
Strength question	3.	4.		
Limitation statement	5.	6.		
Limitation question	7.	8.		

Table 24–2 Supervision Observation Worksheet

Feedback Form: Strength/Limitation Statement/Question	Verbal Behavior	Nonverbal Behavior
Strength statement		
Strength question		
Limitation statement		
Limitation question		

TV contest shows like *Chopped, Next Design Star, American Idol, America's Got Talent, Project Runway,* and *Food Network Challenge* are all the rage. Use the evaluative interaction to explore how individuals respond to appraisals. Describe three responses the contestants from any reality contest show have had to the judges' critiques and what you think about their reaction. If you were the judge (or supervisor) how would you like the contestant (or supervisee) to respond to your review (or feedback)? What type of response would you not tolerate?

_____

_____

_____

_____

How do you react when you are provided with feedback—positively or negatively?

_____

_____

_____

_____

Describe your feelings about being in the role of supervisor.

_____

_____

_____

_____

◻ *Suggestions for Prediction*

Compare and contrast the benefits of oral feedback and written feedback.

_____

_____

_____

_____

A supervisor might organize evaluation around verbal and nonverbal behaviors. Around what other features might a supervisor organize evaluation?

_____

_____

_____

_____

If your ideal supervision style was a vehicle (car, bike, train ...) what kind would it be? Explain your choice.

_____

_____

_____

_____

How can you begin the process of self-critiquing or self-supervision?

_____

_____

_____

_____

What is the procedure in your institution if you have a serious disagreement with your supervisor?

_____

_____

_____

_____

With whom do you talk about a serious disagreement with your supervisor? Complete the statements below, identifying the chain of command you would follow.

If I have a serious disagreement with my supervisor, the first person I should talk to is _____ .

If the issue cannot be resolved, I should talk with _____

_____ .

If I need to take it to the next level, I should then talk to _____

_____ .

ANSWERS

A. The answers to A are shown in **Table 24–3**.

Table 24–3 Supervision Activity Answers

Feedback Form: Strength/Limitation Statement/Question	Verbal Behavior	Nonverbal Behavior	Your Plan for Using This Information to Improve	
			Verbal	Nonverbal
Strength statement	1. g	2. e	I will continue to aim my utterance length at slightly higher than the client's mean length of utterance (MLU). To help myself monitor this, I will do a five-minute online transcription bi-weekly and examine utterance length.	I will make sure I write directions on anything I send home. Making the verb—what he needed to do in the assignment—in bold letters seems to be a useful strategy that I should use more often.
Strength question	3. f	4. h	I felt good about the assessment information. Actually writing a script and practicing it really helped my confidence. I will remember that strategy next time I go to share assessment information.	I never realized that I was pausing and giving more time during book reading. I will try to pause for seven seconds after I make a comment or ask a question during our initial conversation routine next session and see if response accuracy increases for that task.
Limitation statement	5. b	6. a	I cannot believe I did that. I know /p/ and /b/ are cognate pairs—the only difference is in voicing, not place or manner. I will go back to my phonetics text and recheck on characteristics of the phonemes so I do not make this rookie mistake again.	I had not considered wait time as being different across cultures. I'll see if I can find this information on the internet or in my text but I do not remember it ever being addressed in my classes. If I can not find the information, I will go and talk with my supervisor and get additional information and direction.
Limitation question	7. d	8. c	I know I need to slow my rate, especially with this client with fluency goals. I will write "slow" on the top of my data sheet to remind myself.	When we sit side by side, I will make sure her chair is nearer the mirror so I do not block the view for the observers. I will arrange the chairs in this manner before the session.

CHAPTER 25

Group Remediation

THE FOCUS

Group remediation is when a clinician works with two or more clients at the same time. In contrast, individual remediation is working with only one person in a time period. Both group and individual remediation are viable options for provision of speech services to children and adults. Both options have inherent benefits and challenges associated with this difference in the number of clients being treated simultaneously. Since the focus of this chapter is group remediation, a closer examination of its strengths and limitations is appropriate. Having two or more clients involved in a session increases the potential for generalization of skills being practiced into conversational speech, for evaluation of others' speech, and for development of relationships with peers. The group atmosphere often leads to discussion of topics especially relevant to the members as it is introduced and/or sustained by the members. With more people introducing and commenting on topics, the variety of interesting conversations increases. Peers may be able to follow the clinician's model of the best way to interact with another member of the group or simply have a common experience to converse about when the session is completed.

Conversely, having more people involved in a session decreases the potential for individual new learning without awkwardness, for the undivided attention of the clinician, and for the client's active engagement throughout the session. While a clinician might intend to spend an equal amount of the group session with each client, this is rarely accomplished. The client with challenging behaviors, one seated in a chair directly in the clinician's line of sight, or one joyfully demanding attention might in fact be involved with the clinician far more of the session than the predicted percentage (the number of minutes divided by number of clients in the session).

Thus, group remediation challenges clinicians to carefully plan production, listening, and quiet practice (seat work) tasks to fully engage all clients throughout the entire session. It is especially important to remember when planning group remediation that learning can take place in a range of activities that involve speaking, listening, reading, writing, or thinking.

While we cannot identify what will work for your particular group, we offer some suggestions that, when modified, may begin to address your specific needs in conducting your group's remediation.

Consideration 1: Clients coming in one at a time or while the previous group is leaving.

Solutions:

- Have folders all clients pick up as they enter and a worksheet for each to begin and work on until all individuals are present.
- Design an interactive bulletin board where clients complete a matrix (e.g., putting the picture or word from the possible choices into the appropriate spot) or practice their individual generalization stories until you call them to work.
- Use this time for conversation to build relationships, determine interests, carry over targets, and identify additional assessment probes required.

Consideration 2: Group is mixed with varied ages, diagnoses, goals, levels, or physical abilities.

Solutions:

- Have a theme such as endangered species, travel, or an important date in history that connects the session yet allows the versatility for each to address their individual goals.
- Assign each a role such as speaker, time keeper, listening partner, chart recorder, etc., so all are involved in different ways at all times or in a more simplified version, have all members in the group hold up a "thumbs-up" or "thumbs-down" card for all productions.
- Use individual seat work requiring drawing, reading, or writing to focus part of the group while you work with the others.
- Work as a team on a project that incorporates each individual's goals (e.g., a newsletter for families and friends). Partial participation allows all to participate in the project to the level they are able. Setting up alternative goals for individuals promotes participation in the same task as others in the room at a different level or in a different mode or for a different purpose.

Consideration 3: A client disrupts others around him/her.

Solutions:

- Establish and post rules for behavior including turn taking. Rules can include visual symbols or pictures for nonreaders and should be stated in positive terms naming the behavior you desire.

- Establish a token reward system and provide incentives for appropriate behaviors—catch them being good. In the school setting, continue the method the teacher has established for recognizing good behavior.
- Arrange seating to facilitate compliance (i.e., space between people and proximity to the instructor).

THE ACTIVITY

A. Identify whether the action phrase in the following list is a clear strength for group remediation (GrR), individual remediation (InR), or is equally a strength for both group and individual remediation (BothR) by writing the appropriate abbreviation in the space provided before each item. Then provide the rationale for your decisions by completing the *because* portion of the sentence.

1. _____ Addressing goals because _____

_____

_____

2. _____ Generalizing new learning into conversation with a peer

because _____ _____

_____

_____

3. _____ Talking about feelings without embarrassment because

_____

_____

4. _____ Evaluating others' speech because _____

_____

_____

5. _____ Practicing listening skills because _____

_____

_____

6. _____ Having one-on-one time with a clinician because _____

_____

_____

7. _____ Feelings of inclusion because _____

_____

_____

8. _____ Learning a new skill because _____

_____

_____

9. _____ Practicing a skill once learned because _____

_____

_____

10. _____ Making effective use of time because _____

_____

_____

B. While observing a session with two or more clients, estimate the amount of time that each client is spending on producing, listening, quiet practicing (seat work), and off task behaviors by completing **Table 25–1**. Give a descriptor such as shirt color or hair length so you will remember which client is designated as A, B, C, or D. At the end of each 10-minute section, write the approximate number of minutes out of 10 that each client spent on each type of task. Make sure each client's time sums to 10 minutes for each of the segments evaluated. After you complete the data on the task/time for each client, complete the last row of the chart by providing a summary of each person's participation.

Table 25–1 Group Remediation Observation Form

	Descriptor Client A:	Descriptor Client B:	Descriptor Client C:	Descriptor Client D:
First 10 minutes 1. Producing on task 2. Listening on task 3. Quiet practicing on task 4. Off-task behavior				
Second 10 minutes 1. Producing on task 2. Listening on task 3. Quiet practicing on task 4. Off-task behavior				
Third 10 minutes 1. Producing on task 2. Listening on task 3. Quiet practicing on task 4. Off-task behavior				
Fourth 10 minutes 1. Producing on task 2. Listening on task 3. Quiet practicing on task 4. Off-task behavior				
Fifth 10 minutes 1. Producing on task 2. Listening on task 3. Quiet practicing on task 4. Off-task behavior				

(continues)

Table 25-1 Group Remediation Observation Form (continued)

	Descriptor Client A:	Descriptor Client B:	Descriptor Client C:	Descriptor Client D:
Sixth 10 minutes				
1. Producing on task				
2. Listening on task				
3. Quiet practicing on task				
4. Off task behavior				
Actual percentage of involvement (the total number of minutes of producing + listening + quiet practicing divided by the number of minutes in the session).				
Predicted percentage of involvement (the number of minutes in the session divided by number of clients in the session; this should be the same number for each client).				

THE WRAP-UP

◻ *Suggestions for Reflection*

Describe each client's pattern of engagement from your time estimates. Did all clients have similar patterns of on- and off-task behaviors? Why or why not?

_____

_____

_____

_____

Did the clinician appear to have a favorite in the session? What clinician behaviors led you to this decision?

_____

_____

_____

_____

What changes might the clinician make in the plan for next session to modify the patterns you observed?

_____

_____

_____

_____

What additional suggestions could you make based on your observation or personal experience for the three considerations we listed at the end of the focus information?

- Clients coming in one at a time or while the previous group is leaving.

_____

_____

_____

_____

- The group is mixed with varied ages, diagnoses, goals, levels, and physical abilities.

_____

_____

_____

_____

- A client disrupts others around him/her.

_____

_____

_____

_____

◻ Suggestions for Prediction

What additional rating category beyond producing, listening, quiet practicing, and off-task behaviors would you have included? Why?

_____

_____

_____

_____

The clinician is recommending a change from individual to group remediation for a child with fluency errors and an adult with aphasia. Imagine a scenario for each case. Write a justification for the change in treatment from individual to group in both example clients. Include details such as the length of time each had been in individual treatment, their current levels of performance, and the specific advantages for the group placement most relevant to each scenario.

Scenario 1. A child with fluency errors

_____

_____

_____

_____

Scenario 2. An adult with aphasia

_____

_____

_____

_____

ANSWERS

A.

1. BothR. Addressing goals because every session is planned for precisely this reason.

2. GrR. Generalizing new learning into conversation with a peer because peers are actually present in group sessions and generalization would not be as big a step.

3. InR. Talking about feelings without embarrassment because an individual session affords more privacy.

4. GrR. Evaluating others' speech because others would be present and the clinician is providing specific, ongoing evaluation for comparison of each client's personal evaluation. This is a type of incidental learning that can be beneficial in group remediation.

5. GrR. Practicing listening skills because a group session has a variety of people with whom to interact.

6. InR. Having one-on-one time with a clinician because the entire session in individual therapy is one-on-one, but only a portion of the group session is specifically focused on any one individual.

7. GrR. Feelings of inclusion because group sessions can promote camaraderie and shared experiences between peers.

8. InR. Learning a new skill because of the increased individual time available in individual remediation.

9. BothR. Practicing a skill once learned because both afford practice opportunities.

10. BothR. Making effective use of time because both have this potential. How effectively the time is spent depends on the skill of the clinician, not the type of session.

CHAPTER 26

Safety and Security

As clinicians, it is important to understand the safety policies of your clinic. Chances are if you have been to a doctor's appointment in the last few years, you have had to sign a form stating you were given a copy of the policies. The Health Insurance Portability and Accountability Act of 1996, better known as HIPAA, was instituted to ensure clients' privacy. This act states that a person's medical information will not be shared with anyone other than with people to whom the client has agreed to release that information. Clinics must make sure that files are kept in a safe or locked area, that information about a client is kept out of the public's sight, and that information such as reports are sent only to those individuals to whom the client has given permission. In some clinics there are observation rooms. Those observation rooms must remain locked if those rooms are accessible through a public hallway.

Not only are the clinics liable for keeping clients' information private, but any individual working with clients must also follow HIPAA guidelines. For students and clinicians, this means that you are not allowed to openly discuss identifying information about a client. You cannot talk about your clients to a friend or anyone else and use any identifying information such as their name. You may not put identifying information in a document and use it in class or share with anyone unless you have written consent from the client or the client's legal guardians. This proves to be difficult for many students because they want to discuss a client or ask questions to help them better assist the client. You may still talk in general terms about a client or situation, but you may not use any information that could allow that client to be identified.

Chances are, before you were allowed to begin observations, you were required to sign some HIPAA paperwork stating that you agree to the requirements outlined by the act. The penalties for breaking the requirements of the act vary from warnings, to payback issues, to prison time. It is vital that you familiarize yourself with the HIPAA policy of your clinic sites and that you keep these requirements in mind when you enter the workforce.

A different focus of safety and security that is important to remember is your own safety and security. As clinicians, you may be exposed to various situations depending on your work environment. For example, if you work in a hospital or medical setting you will need to have hepatitis B vaccinations or sign a waiver with your facility. It is up to you to familiarize yourself with your site and conditions that you may be exposed to during work. Even in a university clinical setting, you will be exposed to a variety of medical conditions. Sometimes your exposure will be very limited and other times you may get a great deal of exposure. We recommend you explore topics from blood-borne pathogens to tuberculosis as well as be aware of common viruses that may be spread. Washing your hands is your best defense against most airborne bacteria and viruses. In our clinic we have instituted a policy that all clinicians will thoroughly wash their hands between clients and use the antibacterial gel that is provided in each of the rooms at the beginning of a session. Clinicians are also encouraged to have their clients use the gel in the rooms as well. Materials and equipment including table surfaces need to be disinfected after each use. It is important to know and follow safety and security procedures for the well-being of your clients and yourself.

You should familiarize yourself with procedures during various activities. For example, when clinicians are performing oral peripheral exams they should make sure they use gloves. When removing the gloves, turn them inside out as you take them off so that your hands do not touch the outside of the gloves. They should be placed in a biohazard container. You should familiarize yourself with your site's policy on cleaning up bodily fluids. These should always be cleaned immediately, but you may need to follow up with someone at your site to report the incident so more thorough cleaning can be conducted.

THE ACTIVITY

A. Read the following scenarios and determine if HIPAA guidelines are being followed:

Scenario 1. A phone call is made to remind a client of an appointment. After generic answering machine greeting, the following message is left, "Hello, this is Zeta from the Speech and Hearing Clinic. I am calling to remind you that Johnny Turntaker has an appointment here tomorrow for a speech-language evaluation at 10 a.m. Please call us at (999) 999-9999 if you are not going to be able to keep this appointment. We look forward to meeting you and Johnny tomorrow and will have more information regarding Johnny's eligibility for speech/language services following the evaluation."

_____

_____

_____

_____

Scenario 2. A client comes into the clinic and signs in on the sign-in sheet provided at the front desk. When it is time for the appointment, the clinician comes out to the waiting room and calls the client's name.

_____

_____

_____

_____

Scenario 3. Susan's grandmother stops by and wants a copy of Susan's last evaluation. Susan's grandmother is not the legal guardian and her name is not on the release of information, but she brings Susan almost every week to her appointment so a copy of the report is given to her.

_____

_____

_____

_____

Scenario 4. Jack and Diane are discussing their week in the student room. Diane has been struggling with keeping her client interested in the treatment activities, and Jack had the same client last semester. Diane asks Jack for some assistance with this client by saying, "Jack, you know the little girl you had last semester who was working on /r/? I have her this semester, and I was hoping you could give me some idea of the treatment activities she enjoyed."

_____

_____

_____

_____

Scenario 5. An SLP from a local school system calls and wants some information on a child who will be transferring to their school. The father signed a release of information for the school system last week. The SLP would like to discuss the client with the supervisor and would like a copy of the last report.

_____

_____

_____

_____

B. Think about the security of information for the client you just observed. Do you have access to his or her file? What information is important to review before sending out any documents? Where are the files kept? How long can you check the file out? Where are you allowed to review the chart? Write a paragraph describing security of information for this particular client.

_____

_____

_____

Now think about safety for the client you just observed. Do you see any safety hazards? What precautions were taken to make the environment safe? Do you see a biohazard container? Were materials sanitized? Write a paragraph describing safety precautions in place and relevant for this particular client.

_____

_____

_____

While observing, document any situation that occurred that dealt with safety and security of either the client, clinician, or protected information. How was the situation resolved?

_____

_____

_____

_____

THE WRAP-UP

◻ *Suggestions for Reflection*

Why is there such a law as the Health Insurance Portability and Accountability Act?

_____

_____

_____

_____

What are the best practices when it comes to taping clients and reviewing the tapes or using them for instructional purposes in class or in research?

_____

_____

_____

_____

◻ *Suggestions for Prediction*

Imagine you are setting up a private practice office. What resources are available for developing with your HIPAA documents? What options are available with regard to electronic charting?

_____

_____

_____

_____

Why is it important to be aware of possibility of disease exposure in various settings? What are your options for obtaining vaccinations? What are some resources you could use when finding out about exposure?

_____

_____

_____

_____

A.

Scenario 1. This is a violation because with a generic answering machine greeting, the only message you should leave is your name and number for a return phone call.

Scenario 2. Privacy should be maintained. Use of first name is appropriate.

Scenario 3. You are not permitted to release the report. To be in compliance, you may not share the report with anyone not on the release (even if they accompany the client to her sessions).

Scenario 4. This is permissible. No identifying information has been used. Speaking about therapy in general terms is appropriate.

Scenario 5. The release of information should be received before the information is shared.

B.

You should have access to the file, the release of information should be reviewed before sharing any information with anyone, files should be kept in a locked area, you should have to have the file back before the close of business, there are probably designated areas for reviewing charts.

CHAPTER 27

New Learning, Practice, and Generalization

THE FOCUS

In a language therapy session, a client is guided by the clinician through new learning, practice, and generalization. All three components are essential.

1. The clinician uses a variety of teaching strategies to facilitate the client's new learning. Some of the strategies are direct, such as identifying a language rule (e.g., the rule for past tense as when an action already happened, we add an *ed* to the end of the verb). Some strategies for new teaching are indirect, such as staging the scene to make the new learning necessary (e.g., placing desired items out of reach to require a client to demonstrate requesting behavior).

2. Practice allows the client to use the newly targeted skill correctly. The clinician carefully controls difficulty and provides scaffolding or support at a sufficient level to allow the client to practice the skill successfully. A hierarchy of clinician support is commonly used and individualized for the specific client. The hierarchy ranges from minimal-level support such as "Remember our language rule for something that already happened," or "Use your words," through a mid-level support such as, "Put an *ed* on bake to tell me what the girl did yesterday," or "Do you want juice or milk?" to a high level of support such as, "Tell me she baked," or "Say 'juice.'" A clinician gauges the degree of support required to provide the minimal amount of support that still allows the client to be successful in practicing the new learning. Feedback, whether in the form of a natural consequence, a turn, or a verbal comment, etc., is critical.

3. Generalization or carryover involves the extension of what was learned to new items, settings, or partners. The attainment of generalization is the crux of language remediation. A client must be able to use the skill learned and practiced in therapy beyond the session and in a broader fashion that ultimately includes novel language and unique communication partners. Generalization can be encouraged within the session by providing conversation and role-playing opportunities and beyond the session by providing homework.

THE ACTIVITY

A. Identify the degree of support the clinician is providing in the following script by listing MinS for minimal-level support, MidS for mid-level support, or HighS for high-level support in the 15 spaces provided in the last column of **Table 27–1**. The therapy scenarios are based on the classroom teaching method developed and demonstrated by Anita Archer (2008). Check your responses against the answers provided.

AS YOU OBSERVE...

B. While watching the session tally the degree of support the clinician provides by placing a check in the appropriate box (minimal-, mid-, or high-level support). When you have 20 tally marks each for minimal-level support, mid-level support, and high-level support (or the end of the session has arrived), write an example the clinician used for each level.

Minimal-level support:

Example:

_____

_____

_____

_____

Table 27–1 Level of Support Activity Worksheet

Clinician	Children as Group Response (All) or Individual Child Response (Child's Name)	Component of the Session: New Learning Practice Generalization Review	Rating of Clinician Support: MinS MidS HighS
Welcome to language class, Tom, Dick, and Harry. We learned two words that are opposites last time. One of those words was *bottom*. The other word was ___.	No response (all)	Review	1. ___
Miss Smith has you put your name *not at the bottom* of the page but at the ___.	Top (Harry)		2. ___
Harry's got it. We put our name at the ___. The opposite of *top* is ___. *Bottom.*	Top (all) Bottom (Dick)		3. ___
			4. ___
Our opposite words for today are *first* and *last*. Check the board; this word is *first*. This word is ___.	First (all)	New learning	5. ___
Yes, *first. First* means number one, the start, the beginning. Another word for the beginning item is ___.	First (all)		
Yes, *first.* The next word on the board is *last.* This word is ___.	Last (all)		6. ___
Yes, *last. Last* means the end item. Another word for the end is ___.	Last (all)		7. ___
			8. ___

(continues)

Table 27–1 Level of Support Activity Worksheet (continued)

Clinician	Children as Group Response (All) or Individual Child Response (Child's Name)	Component of the Session: New Learning Practice Generalization	Rating of Clinician Support: MinS MidS HighS
Tom, our two words for today are _____ and _____.		Practice	
The top word (on the board) means the same as beginning but it starts with an /f/ sound. This word is _____, Tom.	Beginning and last (Tom)		9. _____
The word on the board that means the same as beginning or start is *first*. This word that means beginning or start is _____.	Start?		10. _____
Practice continues with talk of car races, lining up for recess, and my place in a race if my shoe comes untied and everyone else crosses the finishing line before me.	First (Tom)		11. _____
	Each has at least 10 opportunities to respond individually or in the group.		
Let's look for the words *first* and *last* (pointing to the words on the board) on the directions for the work sheet Miss Smith gave you this morning. Put your finger on the word *first*. Look carefully at our word on the board. Dick, the word is in this line and starts with an *f*. (Nods her head)		Generalization	
	Two point correctly.		12. _____
Now look at the word *last*; it starts with the *l*. Put your finger on the word *last*.	Dick points correctly.		13. _____
Put your finger on the word that tells us what we will do to start.	All point correctly.		14. _____
	All point correctly.		15. _____

Mid-level support:

Example:

_____

_____

_____

_____

High-level support:

Example:

_____

_____

_____

_____

THE WRAP-UP

◻ *Suggestions for Reflection*

Which was the first level of support that you scored 20 examples? Why do you think this level was completed first in this session?

_____

_____

_____

_____

If the purpose of the practice portion of the session is to perform the target correctly, what does a 20 percent accuracy rate suggest to you?

_____

_____

_____

_____

◻ Suggestions for Prediction

Ideally, how much time do *you* think should be spent in each of the three components of new learning, practice, and generalization? What factors are critical to consider when making that determination?

_____

_____

_____

_____

Should generalization activities be included from the beginning of treatment or be reserved for the final step in the treatment process? Support your answer.

_____

_____

_____

_____

ANSWERS

   A.

      1. MinS

      2. MidS

      3. MinS

      4. MidS

5. HighS

6. MidS

7. HighS

8. MidS

9. MinS

10. MidS

11. MidS

12. MinS

13. MidS

14. MidS

15. MinS

REFERENCE

Archer, A. (2008, November). *Getting them all engaged: Inclusive active participation.* Presentation at the American Speech-Language Hearing Association Convention. Chicago, IL.

CHAPTER 28

Session Notes

THE FOCUS

It is important for continuity, tracking change, and reimbursement purposes that accurate and accessible logs of clinical sessions be maintained. A common type of session log is termed the SOAP note. The acronym stands for subjective, objective, assessment, and plan. Subjective information is descriptive and may include observed or reported (by client or family) emotions or behaviors. A statement such as "Mother reported child has been sluggish since the seizure experienced last night," or "Mr. Jones appeared eager to attend and share his completed assignment from last session" is appropriate for the *S* section of the note. Objective information is client performance data from the session. Similar to a behavioral objective, it should include the behavior, condition, and level accomplished. Data statements such as "Mary produced /r/ with 70 percent accuracy (7/10) given modeled words," and "Joe used spontaneous three-word utterances eight times within the 30-minute session" are examples of *O* information. Probing information for nonpractical items that are presented periodically to assess generalization of learning is also common in the *O* section. Assessment information is the clinician's judgment of the meaning or interpretation of the *S* and *O* information. Comparison of present performance demonstrated in this session to past sessions is fitting. Evaluative statements might include, "High accuracy rate with minimal support for the second session at the word level suggests achievement of objective at this level" or "Significant decrease in accuracy rates may be related to client's lack of interest in the materials utilized." The plan incorporates changes based on the *A* statements. Plans may include statements such as, "Level will be raised to phrases" or "New materials that require movement will be introduced."

THE ACTIVITY

A. Use the SOAP note checklist in **Table 28–1** to evaluate the SOAP note of a beginning clinician that follows. Then rewrite the SOAP note. Compare your checklist to the one included under "Answers" and see the rewrite of the log.

Sample Beginning Clinician SOAP Note Concerning the Treatment Session of a College-Aged, Hearing-Impaired Client:

S. I asked the client about her semester. The client talked a lot about being scared to give speeches in her Speech 101 class. She was worried about not talking loud enough, making errors on her "s" and "z" sounds, and saying long words so others could understand them.

O. The client had 50% accuracy on long words she brought to the session. She had 80% accuracy of "s" in isolation. She had 70% accuracy on single-syllable "s" words (drill list). She had 20% accuracy on single syllable "s" words (drill list) used in phrases. She had 20% accuracy of generalization probe of unpracticed words with "s" and "z".

A. She tried hard and did some tasks better than others.

P. Include practice on her speech for Speech 101 class. Keep working on /s/ at word and phrase level.

Rewrite of sample SOAP note:

S

_____

_____

_____

_____

O

_____

_____

_____

_____

Table 28–1 SOAP Note Activity Checklist

Characteristic	Yes Appropriate	Revision Required
1. Is individualized description included under the *S*?		
2. Does the subjective description provide observed or reported information relevant to the treatment?		
3. Does data included under the *O* include behavior, condition, and level accomplished?		
4. If percentages are used, are the number correct/ number of opportunities provided (e.g., 10/20)?		
5. Are all the goals addressed in the session included in either the *S* or *O*?		
6. Is the information under *S* and *O* brought together and evaluated under *A*?		
7. Is current performance compared to previous performance under the *A*?		
8. Does the *P* reflect information under the *A*?		
9. Are changes in objectives, level, clinician support, target items, strategy, etc., identified in the plan?		
10. Is the SOAP note about the client's performance and not the clinician's attempts?		
11. Is writing terminology professional (e.g., *clinician* used [not *I*], *child* used [not *kid*], and person-first language used [not disorder-first language]) and content accurate?		
12. Is writing form correct (e.g., grammar, spelling, and phonetic symbol use), and has the note been proofread?		

A

_____

_____

_____

_____

P

_____

_____

_____

_____

AS YOU OBSERVE...

B. Write a first draft of a SOAP note concerning the session you are observing. Make sure you collect performance data to use in the *O* section. Use the checklist (**Table 28–2**) to evaluate the SOAP note you have written. Make corrections to your first draft of your SOAP note in the margins.

S (subjective)

_____

_____

_____

_____

O (objective)

_____

_____

_____

_____

A (assessment)

_____

_____

_____

_____

P (plan)

_____

_____

_____

_____

Table 28–2 Observation SOAP Note Checklist

Characteristic	Yes Appropriate	Revision Required
1. Is individualized description included under the *S*?		
2. Does the subjective description provide observed or reported information relevant to the treatment?		
3. Does data included under the *O* include behavior, condition, and level accomplished?		
4. If percentages are used, are the number correct/ number of opportunities provided (e.g., 10/20)?		
5. Are all the goals addressed in the session included in either the *S* or *O*?		
6. Is the information under *S* and *O* brought together and evaluated under *A*?		
7. Is current performance compared to previous performance under the *A*?		
8. Does the *P* reflect information under the *A*?		
9. Are changes in objectives, level, clinician support, target items, strategy, etc., identified in the plan?		
10. Is the SOAP note about the client's performance and not the clinician's attempts?		
11. Is writing terminology professional (e.g., *clinician* used [not *I*], *child* used [not *kid*], and person-first language used [not disorder-first language]) and content accurate?		
12. Is writing form correct (e.g., grammar, spelling, and phonetic symbol use), and has the note been proofread?		

THE WRAP-UP

◘ *Suggestions for Reflection*

How is the writing in a SOAP note the same and different from writing you have done in the past?

_____

_____

_____

_____

How did knowing that you would be required to write a SOAP note of a session influence your observation of the session?

_____

_____

_____

_____

◻ *Suggestions for Prediction*

Examine the importance of writing logs and reports to the job of the SLP/ audiologist.

_____

_____

_____

_____

Match to sample means making your writing conform to the example you are provided. Why is it a good idea to get samples of reports and logs from the facility at which you are working?

_____

_____

_____

_____

What factors influence the writing form a training site utilizes?

_____

_____

_____

_____

ANSWER

A. A filled-in checklist is shown in **Table 28–3**.

Rewrite of sample beginning clinician SOAP note:

S. When asked about her semester, the client noted her fear of giving speeches in her Speech 101 class. She was concerned specifically about loudness, articulation of /s and z/ sounds, and production of multisyllable words.

O. The client had 50% accuracy (1/2) on multisyllable words (consciousness and serendipity) she brought to the session. She achieved 80% accuracy (8/10) of /s/ in isolation. She scored 70% accuracy

Table 28–3 SOAP Note Activity Checklist

Characteristic	Yes Appropriate	Revision Required
1. Is individualized description included under the *S*?	Yes	
2. Does the subjective description provide observed or reported information relevant to the treatment?	Yes	
3. Does data under the *O* include behavior, condition, and level accomplished?	Yes	
4. If percentages are used, are the number correct/ number of opportunities provided (e.g., 10/20)?		No
5. Are all the goals addressed in the session included in either the *S* or *O*?	Yes	
6. Is the information under *S* and *O* brought together and evaluated under *A*?		No
7. Is current performance compared to previous performance under the *A*?		No
8. Does the *P* reflect information under the *A*?		No
9. Are changes in objectives, level, clinician support, target items, strategy, etc., identified in the plan?		No
10. Is the SOAP note about the client's performance and not the clinician's attempts?	Generally yes	Exception is initial *S* statement
11. Is writing terminology professional (e.g., *clinician* used [not *I*], *child* used [not *kid*], and person-first language used [not disorder-first language]) and content accurate?	Generally Yes	Some word choices could be more professional
12. Is writing form correct (e.g., grammar, spelling, and phonetic symbol use), and has the note been proofread?		No, phonetic symbols not used

(21/30) on single-syllable /s/ words (drill list). She had 20% accuracy (6/30) on single-syllable /s/ words (drill list) used in phrases and 20% accuracy (2/10) of generalization probe of unpracticed words with /s and z/.

A. The client's homework assignment to identify and bring to the session words she had difficulty producing during the week indicates a focus on multisyllable words containing /s/. These words will be incorporated into practice when work begins on multisyllable levels. She does not appear to notice sound errors on single-syllable words. She has not achieved a high accuracy at the single-word level but she did show a substantial increase from the previous session. Production at the phrase level indicates the need for a step before the independent phrase level or additional support at the phrase level. This is the first session where increase to the probe list has occurred. This generalization to one unpracticed /s/ word and one unpracticed /z/ word is a positive indicator for learning. The speeches from the speech class would provide appropriate practice material and promote generalization.

P. Development of rating scale for loudness, articulation of /s and z/ sounds, and production of multisyllable words to use to monitor training with the material from the Speech 101 class is needed for pre/post measures. Keep procedures at /s/ at word level. A two-word carrier phrase (e.g., one ___, or my ___) should provide the first step towards phrase use. Modifications in directions to focus homework on single-syllable word level are needed.

CHAPTER **29**

Clinician Researcher Connection: Data Collection

THE FOCUS

Clinicians have many opportunities to contribute to the research evidence that shapes practice in the fields of speech pathology and audiology. Single-subject design research, a form of quantitative research, is especially conducive to the examination of clinical questions frequently asked by SLPs. Questions such as *Is this therapy making a change? Which of these two techniques is better for this client?*, or *If I add or subtract this piece of the recommended therapy package, will the resulting therapy be better?* can be answered through systematic data collection within an ABA, multiple baseline, alternating treatments, or interactional form of single subject design (Kearns, 1986). Whether you are collecting data to address specific research questions or to monitor client progress for reporting attainment of therapy goals or quarterly benchmarks in a report card format, the following key elements should be considered:

1. *Operational definition.* Both clinical research and clinical practice become clearer when a written definition of the behavior is developed. This description can include specific examples of scoring and tricky instances of which the rater needs to be especially vigilant. The more specifically the behavior is defined, the more consistently it will be evaluated.

2. *Frequent behavior.* A behavior that occurs infrequently provides few instances to model, treat, or evaluate in either the research or practice venue. Multiple data points are needed to ensure faith in the results. Tasks can be developed, or the environment can often be manipulated to increase the frequency of target behavior occurrence.

3. *Stable baseline.* Clinical researchers and practitioners are interested in the level of the behavior before any attempt to modify is made. The way we know change has occurred is through comparison with initial data. Multiple pretreatment or baseline data measures are gathered until an established starting pattern is determined.

4. *Reliable information.* Both clinical research and clinical practice require that reliable and valid data collection procedures be utilized. Reliability reflects our confidence that the measurement is accurate. Reliable data can be calculated from information scored by different observers scoring the same set of information (interrater reliability) or by a single observer scoring the information multiple times (intrarater reliability). We strive to have the two scores, whether inter- or intrarater, match. The better the match, the more confident we are that the measure is accurate

5. *Representing goals/hypothesis.* The data you are collecting is a reflection of the clinical goal or research hypothesis you have identified. The data needs to reflect all aspects of the goal or hypothesis.

6. *Data collection forms.* The sheet or form developed to collect the data can facilitate the accurate recording of the information as well as the ease of interpretation and retention of the information. Identifying information such as name, date, and explanation of symbols utilized should be included.

7. *Organization.* Once the data have been collected, they need to be arranged in a well-ordered manner. Clinical research typically presents each data point in line graphs. Clinical practice frequently provides the information as percentages or rates of occurrence as summary numerical terms.

8. *Surprise data.* Although researchers and practitioners have formulated a data collection plan, each is aware that unplanned information that also needs to be captured can occur. A single occurrence of a behavior, comment, or note can be telling. Remember to look for and record the unexpected in anecdotal notes or observations.

THE ACTIVITY

I. Identify which of the aforementioned key elements are being addressed in the weak/strong example pairs that follow by placing the name of the key element on the line before the example pair.

1. _____

Weak example of key element: The SLP identified that the client produced the /r/ correctly in 70 percent of the opportunities.

Strong example of key element: The SLP and clinical supervisor independently scored the client's responses and took the number of times they were in agreement divided by the number of agreements and disagreements (see **Table 29–1**) to report a 70 percent correct usage of /r/ with an 80 percent point-to-point reliability between the two independent raters.

2. _____

Weak example of key element: The production of a blend is scored as a cluster reduction if only one of the consonants of the target blend is produced.

Strong example of key element: The production of a blend is scored as a cluster reduction if fewer numbers of consonants are produced than the target blend. Examples of cluster reduction include s/st; t/st; st/str, -/str, k/kl. Note: two consonants next to each other in a multisyllable word such as _doghouse_ or _cupcake_ will be considered to be a blend; /th/, /sh/, and /ch/ are single sounds and not considered to be consonant blends.

Table 29–1 Sample Scoring Reliability

Trial	Clinician's Score as Correct (Yes) or Incorrect (No)	Supervisor's Score as Correct (Yes) or Incorrect (No)	Did the 2 Raters Score the Same (Agreement) or Score Differently (Disagreement)?
1	Yes	Yes	Agreement
2	Yes	Yes	Agreement
3	No	Yes	Disagreement
4	No	No	Agreement
5	Yes	Yes	Agreement
6	Yes	No	Disagreement
7	Yes	Yes	Agreement
8	No	No	Agreement
9	Yes	Yes	Agreement
10	Yes	Yes	Agreement

3. _____

Weak example of key element: The target vocabulary presentation in storybook reading was an effective technique with the client learning 30 new vocabulary words in 12 sessions of treatment.

Strong example of key element: The multiple baseline graphs (**Figure 29–1**) present the learning of 3 sets of 10 vocabulary words when treated sequentially (training began after 3 sessions of baseline for the first set, after 6 sessions of baseline for the second set, and after 9 sessions of baseline for the third set) using a storybook reading technique. Baseline remained stable until treatment on the set of vocabulary words was introduced. Results show clear change corresponded with no treatment/ treatment phases indicating that the learning was the result of the training.

4. _____

Weak example of key element: Greetings were targeted once a session as clinician and client met in the waiting area.

Strong example of key element: A minimum of 10 opportunities for production of greetings per session was achieved through role play, focused book reading, and arranging for individuals to visit the session.

5. _____

Weak example of key element: A blank scrap of paper was used to jot down notes during the session.

Strong example of key element: A consistent recording form was developed to record client data (see **Figure 29–2**).

6. _____

Weak example of key element: The goal has been identified as correct usage of the target phoneme in conversational speech. When 80 percent correct production was achieved in sentences following the clinician's model, the goal was considered met.

Strong example of key element: The goal has been identified as correct usage of the target phoneme in conversational speech. When 80 percent correct production was achieved in sentences following the clinician's model, the goal was considered in progress. When 80 percent correct production was achieved in a speech sample during play, the goal was considered met.

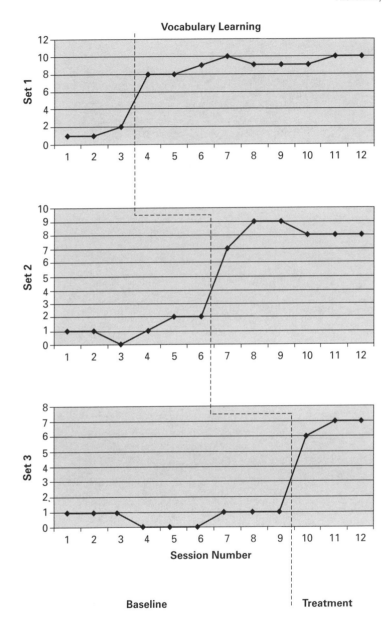

Figure 29–1 **Baseline graphs**

Client Name:_____ _____ Date_____

Recorder:_____

LEVEL OF SUPPORT PROVIDED	ACCURACY
S spontaneous production	+ correct response
M verbal model provided	− incorrect response
C nonverbal cue provided	

Goal/objective:

_____

Target 1: _____

Summary results: ___ / ___   Observation on level of support:

_____

Target 2: _____

Figure 29–2 Datasheets

7. _____

Weak example of key element: After four sessions, the client produced 6/10 non-nasal probe words with appropriate resonance.

Strong example of key element: After four sessions, the client increased his appropriate resonance from a beginning level of 0/10 non-nasal probe words recorded on two consecutive days to a level of 6/10 non-nasal probe words.

Summary results: ___/ ___   Observation on level of support:

_____

Target Item 3: _____

Summary results: ___/ ___   Observation on level of support:

_____

Target Item 4: _____

Summary results: ___/ ___   Observation on level of support:

_____

Target Item 5: _____

Figure 29–2 Datasheets (continued)

8. _____

Weak example of key element: The client completed the assessment tasks and scored in the 30th percentile.

Strong example of key element: The client completed the assessment tasks and scored in the 30th percentile. The client demonstrated several effective strategies during the assessment process. These strategies included repeating the directions he was given, requesting clarification for unfamiliar vocabulary, and asking for feedback at the end of each assessment task.

J. Write a three-to-five-sentence paragraph reflection (thoughts, reactions, and suggestions) on each of the key aspects of data collection. Within each of your eight paragraphs, include examples or expansions based on your current observation.

1. Operational definition:

_____

_____

_____

_____

2. Frequent behavior:

_____

_____

_____

_____

3. Stable baseline:

_____

_____

_____

_____

4. Reliable information:

_____

_____

_____

_____

5. Representing goals/hypothesis:

_____

_____

6. Data collection forms:

_____

_____

_____

7. Organization:

_____

_____

_____

8. Surprise data:

_____

_____

_____

THE WRAP-UP

◻ *Suggestions for Reflection*

Comment on the statement, "Your conclusions are only as accurate as the data on which they are based."

_____

_____

_____

_____

Have you ever used your own personal shorthand when taking notes and had others unable to decipher your meaning or, even more embarrassing, being unable to decode it yourself? Identify three of your personal shorthand notations and their meaning in a key format notation.

_____

_____

_____

_____

Sketch a line graph based on data from the session and then duplicate your sketch using the charting function on your computer (producing computer generated graphs is a useful skill for any clinician). Name three benefits of graphically displayed information in sharing results with clients and families.

Sketch:

_____

_____

_____

_____

◻ Suggestions for Prediction

Complete this analogy: Clinical research is to clinical practice as

_____ is to _____. Explain your choice.

_____

_____

_____

_____

Discuss the pros and cons of developing a task-specific data sheet as compared to using a generic data sheet.

_____

_____

_____

_____

In your opinion, is it best if clinician and researcher are two different individuals or the same individual filling both roles? Make your best argument in support of your position.

_____

_____

_____

_____

ANSWERS

A.

1. Reliable information

2. Operational definition

3. Organization

4. Frequent behavior

5. Data collection form

6. Representing goals/hypothesis

7. Stable baseline

8. Surprise data.

REFERENCE

Kearns, K. (1986). Flexibility of single-subject experimental design. Part II: Design selection and arrangement of experimental phases. _Journal of Speech and Hearing Disorders, 51,_ 204–214.

CHAPTER 30

Putting It All Together

THE FOCUS

This chapter will serve as a general overview of the process of remediation. All clients begin with a referral. The referral can be a self-referral when the client, parent, or family member contacts the center for an appointment. A physician's office or other agency may make a referral for diagnosis or intervention. Almost all insurance policies require a referral from a physician, so if the client is interested in filing an insurance claim, either the client or your facility will be responsible for getting the order from the physician. After the initial referral is made, it is important to determine if a diagnostic is needed (to determine the speech/language/hearing disorder) or if the client has had a recent evaluation and needs to go directly into treatment. Many times, speech-language pathologists and audiologists will do a quick screening, even if a recent evaluation was completed, to make sure there have been no changes with the client or to verify that the goals are still relevant. Baseline data will be gathered to determine exactly how the client is performing on the goals and determine if goals need to be added, modified, or deleted.

After baseline data have been established, it is time to plan the treatment session. Make sure you have activities that are related to the goal. You will also need to know information such as whether the client is on target developmentally, the client's age, any interests of the client that you can incorporate into your session, whether you will use a thematic unit or use various activities (remember you can always use activities more than once with or without modification), and whether there are any physical limitations or other limitations to consider. It is always wise to overplan or have more activities than you anticipate you will need, rather than to underplan.

Remember, you will need to keep data during the session in order to complete your treatment note.

Once you have your treatment session planned, it is time to set up your room. When setting up your room, consider the flow of your activities and if you need to have things out of sight or away from the client. You want to be able to go from one activity to another without a lot of down time, but you may be in a situation that provides too much stimulation when all the materials are within reach for the client. Materials should also be picked up at the conclusion of an activity before another set of materials is introduced. As the clinician, you can use the transition from one activity to another to work on goals. Use every opportunity available to work on goals, such as when you greet the client, when wrapping up the session, or when talking to family members. There are numerous opportunities to work on objectives and goals.

When wrapping up the session, consider having activities that the client can take with him to complete before his next visit. You may want to have information that can be given to family members to learn more about a disorder or a treatment procedure. You may want to develop a tracking sheet that could be used by the client or family so they can document when the client is meeting the target and when the client is struggling. There are many materials that can be given to the client and family members to make sure the client is successful outside the therapy room. Careful consideration of the speech/language difficulty level of these materials will help ensure that the time spent will be goal focused and beneficial.

Following the session, you will need to complete your treatment note. If a formal note is not required, you may want to make sure the data is clearly labeled so you can refer to it in order to plan for the next session. Paperwork is a part of therapy that, when done correctly, can make your life much easier and your therapy more productive. Now, sit back and smile and start thinking of the incredible things you can plan for next time!

THE ACTIVITY

A. Without looking back at the focus material provided, list at least 10 steps that occur in the remediation process in order.

1. _____   6. _____

2. _____   7. _____

3. _____   8. _____

4. _____   9. _____

5. _____   10. _____

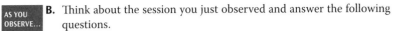

B. Think about the session you just observed and answer the following questions.

1. What are the goals/objectives that were targeted during the session?

_____

_____

_____

_____

2. What activities were used to target the goals/objectives?

_____

_____

_____

_____

3. Come up with one additional activity to target one of the goals/ objectives.

_____

_____

_____

_____

4. Did the clinician keep all activities within sight, or were some put away? Why did this work or not work?

_____

_____

_____

_____

5. Were there activities given to the client/family members at the end of the session?

_____

_____

_____

_____

6. Did the clinician have more activities than were used? Did the clinician run out of activities?

_____

_____

_____

_____

■ *Suggestions for Prediction*

Talk with the clinician following the session. Discuss how much time was spent preparing for the session. Discuss how the clinician uses the data taken during the session to help complete the paperwork and plan for the next session.

_____

_____

_____

_____

If a family member was with the client, do you think the family member has a good understanding of what is going on in therapy and how she can assist the client meet his goals outside therapy? Why or why not?

_____

_____

_____

_____

■ *Suggestions for Prediction*

Do you think it will take less time to plan sessions after you have more experience either as a clinician or with a client? Why or why not?

_____

_____

_____

_____

How can you keep sessions engaging for the client? How can you modify activities or reintroduce them in therapy?

_____

_____

_____

_____

How would your list of steps you recorded previously be modified if you were doing therapy in a collaboration model in a child's classroom or group therapy in a nursing home facility?

_____

_____

_____

_____

ANSWERS

A.

1. Referral

2. Determine diagnosis or screening

3. Gather baseline data

4. Goal writing or modification

5. Write treatment plan

6. Set up environment (room)

7. Gather materials

8. Deliver your treatment

9. Share with family

10. Write session notes

CHAPTER 31

The Clinician I Want to Become

THE FOCUS

As you near the end of your required clinical observation hours, surely some of your questions about the clinical process have been addressed. However, there are bound to be questions still unanswered. Two very individual questions lurking in the minds of many observers likely center on, "Do I possess the characteristics of a model clinician?" and "What kind of clinician will I be?"

The knowledge, skills, and dispositions of an ideal clinician can take many forms. Knowledge reflects access to and understanding of information. Knowledge required to perform as an outstanding SLP includes but is not limited to the knowledge of theoretical underpinnings of the profession, the knowledge of the many disorders associated with our field, the knowledge of what constitutes ethical behavior, and the knowledge of the research literature. Skills refer to application or performance of practice. There is a component of both science and art to the practice of speech therapy and audiology. No cookbook is possible because individual factors are always operating. Some of the skills necessary to the SLP include but are by no means limited to interviewing techniques, test administration, designing structured tasks, analyzing language samples, performing therapy techniques, collecting data, problem solving, and self-evaluating. Finally, the term *disposition* reflects those often-elusive concepts of attitudes or beliefs. The belief in the rights of the individual to receive appropriate services, the belief that families know their members best, and the belief that the communication solutions need to address the individual but also their communication partners and situations all shape the clinician's practice behaviors.

You have probably observed some impressive sessions, some ordinary sessions, and some less-than-stellar sessions. You are beginning to discern those characteristics you wish to refine and develop in yourself in order to pattern yourself after those clinicians who performed truly impressive therapy. Self-reflection is the next step in becoming the best clinician you can be.

THE ACTIVITY

   A. To help you clarify the characteristics of your ideal clinician, develop a list of adjectives that reflect your ideal clinician. Write a characteristic beginning with each letter of the alphabet. Select your top five characteristics and self-evaluate your possession of these vital attributes in **Table 31–1**. Compare your list to the one we developed. Feel free to keep your adjectives or replace some of yours with the ones we compiled. We really struggled with an adjective for *x* and took some creative license to fill in that space.

Table 31–1 Self-Rating Characteristics Worksheet

My Top Five Characteristics	Self-Rating of Your Ownership of This Characteristic 1 = below average; 2 = average; 3 = above average
1.	
2.	
3.	
4.	
5.	

A is for _____   N is for _____

B is for _____   O is for _____

C is for _____   P is for _____

D is for _____   Q is for _____

E is for _____   R is for _____

F is for _____   S is for _____

G is for _____   T is for _____

H is for _____   U is for _____

I is for _____   V is for _____

J is for _____   W is for _____

K is for _____   X is for _____

L is for _____   Y is for _____

M is for _____   Z is for _____

B. To help you address the question, "What kind of clinician will I be?" write a story of how you imagine your first therapy session as the student clinician in charge. Use the stems and word choice items provided below each stem to help develop your story. Select as many of the word choices as you wish to finish the sentence but for each chosen you must complete the *because* phrase that follows.

Once upon a time, there was a speech-language-hearing therapy student. That student therapist was me on the first day I worked with my first client for the first time.

I arrived

- 30 minutes early because _____

_____

- 10 minutes early because _____

_____

◆ as the client walked in the door because _____

_____

◆ late because _____

_____

◆ (writer's choice) _____because

_____

I prepared for the session by reading the client's file/chart to determine

◆ the client's age because _____

_____

◆ my client's name because _____

_____

◆ her parent's name because _____

_____

◆ her diagnosis because _____

_____

◆ her dynamic or structured task results because _____

_____

◆ her formal test results because _____

_____

◆ (writer's choice) _____because

_____

◆ I also prepared by making an appointment and going to see my supervisor with _____

_____

- nothing but a look of confusion on my face because

  _____

- a tentative plan of my session because _____

  _____

- an apology for having no plan due to computer/printer troubles because _____

  _____

- a copy of the client's confidential file that I made to allow me to plan at home when the office was closed because

  _____

- (writer's choice) _____because

  _____

I experienced *lots* of emotions waiting for the client to arrive. I felt

- happy because _____

  _____

- confident because _____

  _____

- scared because _____

  _____

- sick because _____

  _____

- thrilled because _____

  _____

- numb because _____

  _____

- ◆ (writer's choice) _____because

  _____

The session had many positive aspects. These strengths included

- ◆ organization because _____

  _____

- ◆ relationship building because _____

  _____

- ◆ fun and functional activities because _____

  _____

- ◆ sticking to the plan because _____

  _____

- ◆ clear data collection because _____

  _____

- ◆ probing for where to move for the next session because ____

  _____

- ◆ parent/spouse involvement because _____

  _____

- ◆ (writer's choice) _____ because

  _____

Although I was proud of my first session, there were a few limitations that I need to address. The things I would like to improve on next time include

- ◆ my use of specific feedback because_____

  _____

+ remembering to take data/ record information because _____

_____

+ taking the time to talk with significant others because_____

_____

+ having more ideas planned because _____

_____

+ including things to extend the session for the days until we meet again (homework) because _____

_____

+ having considered what I would do for disruptive or off-task behaviors because _____

_____

+ having materials that are more age appropriate because _____

_____

+ (writer's choice) _____because

_____

This session was uniquely mine. My personal touch showed in

+ (writer's choice) _____ because

_____

I learned about being the kind of clinician I want to be from those individuals who allowed me to observe them. The clinician I would most like to thank for being a positive role model is _____ because _____.

Note: Consider writing or e-mailing the individual you have identified as a role model to thank him/her one more time.

THE WRAP-UP

◻ *Suggestions for Reflection*

Connect the characteristics you identified and the clinical observations you have made today. Describe the behaviors observed that reflect some of your identified characteristics.

_____

_____

_____

_____

Visualize yourself as an SLP. Write three sentences describing your visualization.

_____

_____

_____

_____

◻ *Suggestions for Reflection*

Identify two knowledge pieces, two skills, and two dispositions that you have learned that are important to SLPs.

Knowledge 1 _____

Knowledge 2 _____

Skill 1 _____

Skill 2 _____

Disposition 1 _____

Disposition 2 _____

Name two knowledge pieces, two skills, and two dispositions about which you are still a bit unclear. Identify a plan to bring clarity to these points.

Knowledge 1 _____

Knowledge 2 _____

Skill 1 _____

Skill 2 _____

Disposition 1 _____

Disposition 2 _____

Your plan to gain clarity: _____

_____

_____

_____

ANSWERS

A. While many adjectives can fit the letter, here are some we think are appropriate.

A is for adaptable	*N* is for nurturing
B is for bright	*O* is for organized
C is for caring	*P* is for passionate
D is for determined	*Q* is for questioning
E is for enthusiastic	*R* is for reflective
F is for functional	*S* is for sincere
G is for genuine	*T* is for thoughtful
H is for honest	*U* is for upbeat
I is for inquisitive	*V* is for versatile
J is for just	*W* is for wise
K is for knowledgeable	*X* is for xenophobic phobic
L is for lively	*Y* is for youthful
M is for meticulous	*Z* is for zany

CHAPTER 32

Your Turn

THE FOCUS

The chapters in this book have provided you as the clinical observer with opportunities to review a snippet of information ("The Focus"), demonstrate understanding of the reviewed material (first step in "The Activity"), apply this knowledge to the observation of a session (next step in "The Activity"), and reflect on what you observed and connect your thoughts to clinical issues ("The Wrap-Up"). The content of each chapter aimed to be clinically relevant, representative of information available in your pregraduate level classes, and related to an observable facet seen across clients, clinicians, and practicum sites. While the text explored an aspect of each of the big nine and supplemental areas of remediation and presented across area clinical practice instruction, it is just a beginning. Many other focuses, activities, and wrap-ups could be developed based on scope of practice within the field, theoretical influences, and personal passions. Our belief that this is *your* workbook and that *you* should have a hand in developing the content has resulted in the inclusion of this final chapter. We want you to take your turn and write your own chapter as a culminating activity for this workbook. The completion of the information that follows will get you started. Enjoy the freedom and creativity inherent in this activity as you strive to produce something for which you feel a pride of accomplishment.

THE ACTIVITY

A. Determine what additional topic you will choose as your focus. We suggest you consider specific diagnostic categories such as childhood apraxia, Down syndrome, or laryngectomy; specific-age related groupings such as infants, adolescents, or elderly; or specific settings such as preschool classroom, home, or nursing home; or specific issues you identified from your hours of observation. But the choices are endless, so select something you deem to be a valuable addition.

Topic: _____

_____

Write several paragraphs that refresh the reader on the topic. Include an overview, essential vocabulary, and at least one emphasis or key point. Expand the topic with examples to illustrate your point(s). To help in the development of the paragraphs, identify the factors listed.

Three key vocabulary terms with definitions:

Term 1 _____ Definition _____

_____

Term 2 _____ Definition _____

_____

Term 3 _____ Definition _____

_____

Main point(s) you wish to emphasize: _____

_____

because _____

_____

Example 1 to illustrate point: _____

_____

Example 2 to further expand or clarify point: _____

_____

Your personal connection, belief, or suggestion: _____

_____

Put all the aforementioned together and write the focus:

_____

_____

_____

_____

_____

_____

_____

_____

_____

_____

B. Once you have a focus section written, develop an interesting way to test your reader's facilitation with the content information presented. This will be the initial portion of the activity section. Select the format such as definitions, sets of true/false statements, matching, etc., you will use. What format fits with the focus material you have written? What format did you find most useful or enjoyable from the other chapters? Once you select the format, develop numerous items in that format to have your readers complete. Have you addressed your previously identified main point(s)? Have you allowed for practice of new ways of organizing the material? Have you related the content to clinically observable behaviors? Make sure to include directions for what the reader is to do. Complete an answer section and set it apart from the rest of the material with its own heading. To help in the development of the knowledge check activity, identify the factors that follow:

Format(s) chosen to test knowledge from focus material:

_____

because _____

_____

Directions for completion of task(s): _____

_____

_____

_____

Five items for inclusion:

1. _____

2. _____

3. _____

4. _____

5. _____

Answers to the items:

1. _____

2. _____

3. _____

4. _____

5. _____

C. The next part of the activity section should promote observation during an actual session. This needs to be broad enough to accommodate a wide range of observational possibilities. The reader might not be in a similar setting to you or might not have similar past experiences. Just as in the first part of the activity section, you need to select a format, but this format should provide an organized piece for the reader to complete during the observation. Formats we found useful included charts, question sets, and data collection sheets. Provide directions and space for your readers to record their observations. To help in the development of the relevant observation activities, identify the following factors:

Format(s) chosen to test knowledge from focus material:

_____

because _____

_____

Directions for completion of task(s): _____

_____

_____

_____

Form for reader to complete:

D. The final section for you to write is the wrap-up. Here you get to help stimulate the readers' thinking by asking questions that promote examination, application, evaluation, synthesis, analysis, and/or integration. The reflection questions center on what was discovered during the observation or completion of the activities, while the prediction questions center on going beyond what you saw or did and forecasting their future application. This is really about helping the reader move beyond the concrete into the abstract and move from the present to the future. To help in the development of the extension questions, identify the factors listed that follow.

Write one question that promotes each of the behaviors listed below.

Question promoting examination or link to the reader:

_____

_____

_____

_____

Question promoting application or use in an example or scenario:

_____

_____

_____

_____

Question promoting evaluation or identification of strengths and weaknesses:

_____

_____

_____

_____

Question promoting synthesis or connecting with other learning:

_____

_____

_____

_____

Question promoting analysis or breakdown into components or comparison
and contrast:

_____

_____

_____

_____

Question promoting integration or building to a new whole:

_____

_____

_____

_____

Select the best questions you wrote and modify them to correspond to the
reflections and predictions grouping.

Suggestions for reflection:

_____

_____

_____

_____

Suggestions for predictions:

_____

_____

_____

_____

Before you finish your turn as the chapter author, do a last check for accuracy of information, use of person-first language, correct grammar, and precise punctuation and spelling.

Do not be afraid to seek peer or instructor reviews of your chapter. Plan time to polish and rewrite to conclude a successful final product.

THE WRAP-UP

◻ *Suggestions for Reflection*

What do you see as the strengths and weaknesses of your chapter? (Note, this is an evaluation question.)

Name a strength: _____

_____

Name a limitation: _____

_____

What are two ways your observations influence your writing of the chapter? (Note this is a synthesis question.)

1. _____

_____

2. _____

_____

What song title or song lyrics best express your writing of the chapter? (Note, this is an examination question.)

_____

_____

_____

_____

◼ *Suggestions for Prediction*

Why is it important that you be able to direct your own observation? (Note, this is an integration question.)

_____

_____

_____

_____

What skills did you use in writing your chapter that will be important to you as a practicing SLP? (Note, this is an analysis question.)

_____

_____

_____

_____

Observation Log

Name:_____

Instructions: Enter each observation you complete in **Table A–1**. For each observation, complete a different row in the table. Record the date of your observation in column 1, the chapter from this book that you filled out in conjunction with the observation in column 2, the time you observed in 15-minute increments (if you observed 60 minutes, record 1 hour; if 45 minutes, record 0.75 hours; if 30 minutes, record 0.50 hours; and if 15 minutes, record 0.25 hours) in column 3, and a running total of hours you have completed in column 4. In the last column ask your supervisor or Certificate of Clinical Competence (CCC) clinician you are observing to verify the length of your observation by signing his or her name and recording his or her American Speech-Language-Hearing Association certification number.

Table A–1 Clinical Observation Log

Date Day/Month/Year	Book Chapter Completed	Hours Observed	Running Total of Hours Observed	Supervisor/CCC Clinician Signature ASHA Number

ASHA = American Speech-Language-Hearing Association; CCC = Certificate of Clinical Competence

Index